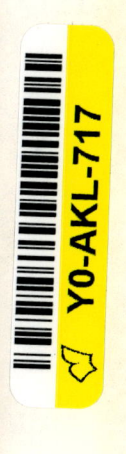

OCCUPATIONAL MEDICINE

HEALTH CARE ECONOMICS AND TECHNOLOGY SERIES

- **Investor-Owned Hospitals and Their Role in the Changing U.S. Health Care System**, by Ekaterini Siafaca, with a Preface by Michael D. Bromberg, Executive Director, Federation of American Hospitals.

- **Medical Product Liability: A Comprehensive Guide and Sourcebook**, Edited by Duane Gingerich.

- **Occupational Medicine: Surveillance, Diagnosis and Treatment**, by the Research Staff of F&S Press, with Michael H. Turk.

- **Medical Diagnostic Imaging Systems: Technology and Applications**, Edited by Betty Hamilton, M.A., with contributions by James A. Patton, Ph.D.; Steven E. Harms, M.D.; and William R. Hendee, Ph.D.

- **Health Maintenance Organizations: Opportunities and Problems**, by Joan Z. Bernstein, Lucy Reed Harris and the Research Staff of F&S Press.

- **Ambulatory Health Care: Models for Development**, by Deborah K. Mullaney.

- **Medical Technology and Government Research: Key Trends in Medical Devices, Instrumentation and Diagnostics Research.**

OCCUPATIONAL MEDICINE
Surveillance, Diagnosis and Treatment

by
The Research Staff of
F&S Press, with
Michael H. Turk

Published by
F&S Press
New York
A Division of Frost & Sullivan, Inc.

Distributed in the U.S. by
Ballinger Publishing Company
Cambridge, Massachusetts
A Subsidiary of Harper & Row, Publishers, Inc.

Copyright © 1982 by F&S Press, a division of Frost & Sullivan, Inc., 106 Fulton Street, New York, NY, 10038. All rights reserved. No part of this publication may be reproduced, stored in a retrieval system, or transmitted in any form or by any means, electronic, mechanical, photocopy, recording or otherwise, without the prior written consent of the publisher.

Printed in the United States of America

First Printing

International Standard Book Number: 0-86621-005-9

Library of Congress Cataloging in Publication Data
Main entry under title:

Occupational medicine.

(Health care economics and technology series)
Bibliography: p.
Includes index.
1. Medicine, Industrial. I. Turk, Michael H.
II. F & S Press. III. Series.
RC963.02   616.9'803   82-5132
ISBN 0-86621-005-9   AACR2

Distributed by Ballinger Publishing Company, 54 Church Street, Cambridge, MA 02138.

Contents

List of Tables	vii
Introduction	3
1. The Political Background: A Legislative History of OSHA	7
2. Environmental Factors in Occupationally Induced Diseases	19
3. Chemical Substances Classified as Major Hazards	29
4. Environmentally Induced Diseases and Disorders	53
5. Techniques in Identifying Harmful Environments	65
6. Medical Surveillance	69
7. Regulation, Legislation, and Research	83
8. Diagnostic and Screening Programs, Equipment and Techniques	103
9. The Occupational Medicine Marketplace	143
10. Suppliers of Products and Services	203
Appendix A: Regional Offices of OSHA	215
Appendix B: Frost & Sullivan Occupational Medicine Questionnaire	217
Appendix C: List of Companies and Institutions that Have Contributed to the Survey	221
Bibliography	227
Index	231

List of Tables

1. Health Effects of Nonionizing Radiation — 24
2. Cancer Causing Substances — 32
3. Substances Causing Eye and Skin Irritation — 51
4. Agents Suspected of Causing Lung Cancer — 55
5. Agents Causing Transient and Permanent Respiratory Disorders — 59
6. Hazardous Substances Affecting Reproductive Function — 60
7. Agents Suspected of Causing Cardiovascular Disorders — 62
8. Agents Causing Central Nervous System Disorders — 63
9. Agents that May Cause Liver Damage — 64
10. Agents that May Cause Kidney Damage — 64
11. Estimated 1977 National Occupational Safety and Health Work Force by Industry and Basic Area — 72
12. Survey Respondents by Professional and Employment Status — 73
13. Federal Agency Support for Environmental Health Research and Related Programs — 86
14. National Institute for Occupational Safety and Health: Obligations by Object Class — 87
15. National Institute for Occupational Safety and Health: Direct and Reimbursable Obligations by Selected Program — 88
16. National Institute of Environmental Health Sciences—1979 and 1980 Budget by Program and Mechanism — 94
17. Medical Surveillance Regimens as Reported by All Survey Respondents — 105
18. Summary of Number and Percent of Plants and Employees in Plants Covered By Special Medical Services—All Industries — 106

LIST OF TABLES

19. Performer of Medical Screening and Medical Equipment in Place as Reported by Survey Respondents — 107
20. Equipment and Techniques in Which New Developments Are Encouraged by the Respondents to the F&S Survey — 108
21. Exposure Hazards that Require Lung Function Tests — 111
22. Number and Percent of Plants and Employees in Plants Covered by Periodic Pulmonary Function Tests for Employees — 112
23. Substances in the Workplace Requiring X-ray Testing of Workers — 115
24. Number and Percent of Plants and Employees in Plants Covered by Periodic Chest X-rays for Employees — 116
25. Number and Percent of Plants and Employees in Plants Covered by Periodic Audiometric Examinations for Employees — 120
26. Substances Requiring Clinical Laboratory Tests — 124
27. Blood Tests Available to Detect Dangerous Exposures to Workplace Hazards — 127
28. Number and Percent of Plants and Employees in Plants Covered by Periodic Blood Tests for Employees — 128
29. Urine Tests Available to Detect Dangerous Exposures to Workplace Hazards — 131
30. Number and Percent of Plants and Employees in Plants Covered by Periodic Urine Tests for Employees — 132
31. Number and Percent of Plants and Employees in Plants Covered by Periodic Ophthalmological Examinations for Employees — 138
32. Estimated Number of People by Industry Exposed to Hazards in Facilities that Do Not Provide Medical Examinations of Any Type — 145
33. Number of Establishments and Total Employees by Industry Groups — 146
34. Number of Establishments by Industry and Special Features — 146
35. Number of Plants and Employees in Plants in the Services Sector — 147
36. Industry Distribution of Survey Respondents—Manufacturing, Mining, and Construction — 148
37. Industry Distribution of Survey Respondents—Utilities, Financial, and Other Services — 149
38. Geographic Distribution of Survey Respondents—Manufacturing, Mining, and Construction — 150
39. Geographic Distribution of Survey Respondents—Utilities, Financial, and Other Services — 152
40. Distribution of Survey Respondents by Size of Establishment — 153
41. Ranking of Hazardous Industries — 154
42. Manufacturing Employment by Industry Type — 155
43. Number of Manufacturing Establishments by Size — 156
44. Number of All Employees of the Manufacturing Industries by Size of Establishment — 158

45.	Number of Production Workers in the Manufacturing Industries by Size of Establishment	160
46.	Summary of Number and Percent of Plants and Employees Covered by Special Medical Services—Manufacturing	162
47.	Number and Percent of Plants and Employees in Plants that Have a Formally Established Health Unit—Manufacturing	163
48.	Number and Percent of Plants and Employees in Plants Covered by the Regular Recording of Health Information about New Employees	165
49.	Number and Percent of Plants and Employees in Plants Covered by Preplacement Physical Examinations of Employees	167
50.	Number and Percent of Plants and Employees in Plants Covered by Periodic Medical Examinations	169
51.	Testing Regimen as Reported by Respondents in the Food and Tobacco Industry	172
52.	Testing Regimen as Reported by Respondents in the Textile Industry	173
53.	Testing Regimen as Reported by Respondents in the Paper and Wood Products Industries	175
54.	Testing Regimen as Reported by Respondents in the Chemicals Industry	177
55.	Summary of Number and Percent of Plants and Employees in Plants Covered by Special Medical Services—Chemicals Industry	178
56.	Testing Regimen as Reported by Respondents in the Petroleum and Coal Industry	180
57.	Testing Regimen as Reported by Respondents in the Primary Metals Industry	182
58.	Testing Regimen as Reported by Respondents in the Fabricated Metals Industry	183
59.	Testing Regimen as Reported by Respondents in the Machinery, Except Electrical, Industry	185
60.	Testing Regimen as Reported by Respondents in the Electrical and Electronic Industry	186
61.	Testing Regimen as Reported by Respondents in the Transportation Equipment Manufacturers Industry	188
62.	Testing Regimen as Reported by Respondents in the Utilities Industry	190
63.	Summary of Number and Percent of Plants and Employees in Plants Covered by Special Medical Services—Utilities	191
64.	Testing Regimen as Reported by Respondents in the Banking and Insurance Industries	192
65.	Summary of Number and Percent of Plants and Employees in Plants Covered by Special Medical Services—Finance, Insurance, and Other	194

LIST OF TABLES

66. Historic and Estimated Total Value of Health Screening Services in Occupational Medicine for the 1974-1989 Period ... 198
67. Historic and Estimated Dollar Markets of Medical Equipment and Devices Acquired by Industry-Based Health Departments in the 1974-1989 Period ... 199
68. Decision Makers in the Operation of a Company Screening Program ... 202
69. Product Manufacturers ... 204
70. Service Providers ... 210

OCCUPATIONAL MEDICINE

Introduction

There is an undisputed link between environment and health. This link becomes even more pronounced in the case of industrial workers who are often relentlessly exposed to an unnatural atmosphere created by the manufacturing processes carried out at their place of work.

There are about 80 million workers in the United States. Approximately 57 million of these, employed by 4100 business establishments, are covered by the Occupational Safety and Health Act. Annually about seven million workers are injured in work-related mishaps and of these 14,000 die and 2.5 million are disabled. The National Institute for Occupational Safety and Health (NIOSH) estimates that there are 390,000 new cases of occupational illness annually (excluding accidental injuries) and 100,000 deaths per year can be attributed to occupationally induced diseases.

What is considered to be an occupational injury or illness? As defined by the Occupational Safety and Health Administration (OSHA), an occupational injury is any physical injury, such as a cut, fracture, sprain, or traumatic amputation that results from a work-related accident or from exposure involving a single incident in the work environment. An occupational illness is any abnormal condition or disorder, other than one resulting from an occupational injury, caused by exposure to environmental factors associated with employment. Included are acute and chronic illnesses that may be caused by inhalation, absorption, ingestion, or direct contact with toxic substances.

Occupationally induced diseases result from negligence, ignorance, and abuse. Abuse occurs when employers place uninformed workers in dangerous environments even though the employers themselves are fully cognizant of the hazard. It is hoped that cases of industrial abuse, such as the Kepone incident, will be relatively rare because of stringent government regulations and the specter of huge liability payments. Negligence occurs when employers fail to assess the risk presented to workers engaged in certain plant activities. There have been attempts to remedy this problem through regulations requiring that employers maintain records regarding employee health status and work environment standards. Ignorance reflects unknown hazards, such as multiple exposure effects, long-range effects, and predisposition. This latter stumbling block in ensuring a healthy work environment will be removed only after the undertaking of extensive and costly research.

The effects of the environment on human health and disease are not readily discernible. Occupational medicine is a very inexact science and its problems are compounded by the fact that its practitioners are operating on a thin ledge between health and economic priorities. In the last few years great strides have been made in identifying potentially hazardous materials and environments. Currently, strict environmental monitoring standards are in place in most manufacturing plants to insure that the atmospheric concentration of hazardous emissions does not exceed a minimum acceptable level. Although the advent of environmental monitoring has been a great step forward in this field, it is not enough to eliminate all health hazards. It is presently believed that environmental monitoring must be combined with medical surveillance to ensure the absence of serious health hazards in the environment.

In order to begin to provide adequate protection against occupationally induced diseases, one must identify all potentially toxic substances that come in contact with workers. This is a monumental task and will not easily be completed. However, many toxic substances have been identified, and regulations have been promulgated to control workers' exposure to such potentially hazardous materials. Each substance identified has a different effect on the health of the worker, as is described in the following pages of this book.

Most large manufacturers engaging in operations that create potentially hazardous environments for their employees have on their staffs industrial hygienists and physicians specializing in industrial medicine. Actually, many have large staffs specifically assigned to developing record-keeping techniques for the monitoring and evaluation of any employee health problems which may be related to the work environment. However, the value of in-plant monitoring and medical screening of workers in order to identify potentially hazardous environments is often hampered by the lack of shared standards among employers and the absence of a national policy. Most of the health testing performed today is anecdotal and episodic, since it is often complaint related. However, in many industries and within many companies, both large and small, medical surveillance has become a way of life. The future will undoubtedly see the further standardization of medical examinations concerned with occupational health and safety.

It must be emphasized that this study is only concerned with occupational disease hazards and not with work-related accidents or injuries, which may be better avoided by increased employee education and employers' adherence to regulatory guidelines. Medical hazards, on the other hand, are elusive, and current environmental controls have not provided adequate employee protection. The aim of this report therefore is to define the need for the medical surveillance, diagnosis, and treatment of industrial and other workers and not to itemize all the potential hazards of the working environment. To this end, we concentrate on the current status of employee screening, testing, and diagnostic programs sponsored by industry to ensure workers' well-being. Medical surveillance of the population at risk is recommended, and, indeed, current federal regulations lean toward making some kind of medical surveillance mandatory. Periodic monitoring of employee health does help to provide early detection of potential workplace hazards, and these hazards are further identified by analyzing epidemiological data. In short, our aim is to report on the general practice of preventive medicine in occupational settings.

Environmental monitoring and adherence to lower limits of pollutant concentrations in the environment as mandated by the Environmental Protection Agency (EPA) or OSHA is the responsibility of the safety engineering personnel employed by corporations. Monitoring for air pollutants in the workplace is carried out extensively in most industries and is beyond the scope of this study.

A discussion of the procedures for testing substances to identify those that are toxins and to establish their effect on human health, as performed by both government and industry, is also beyond the scope of this study. The Toxic Substances Control Act (TOSCA) requires that manufacturers pretest new substances for toxicity both for short-term and low-dose long-term effects. Such evaluations are usually carried out in special laboratories by trained scientists, often specialists in toxicology.

Many of the findings and conclusions presented in this study are based on a special survey conducted by Frost & Sullivan (F & S) in 1979. A three-page questionnaire (see Appendix B) was mailed to the 5887 members of the American Occupational Medicine Association. The mailing list included: industrial and occupational physicians, registered and licensed practical nurses in the occupational medicine area, industrial hygienists, and other allied professionals. Altogether 554 replies were received. Of these, 486 represented partially or fully completed questionnaires and form the basis of the field data in this report.

The replies came from various professionals from many industries throughout the nation (see Tables 12, 36, and 37). A list of contributors to the survey is found in Appendix C.

The results of the survey are presented in several sections of this work, arranged by subject matter. Also, these data are juxtaposed against a survey of the marketplace conducted by NIOSH in the 1972-74 period. These two surveys offer an excellent means of identifying changes in the practice of occupational medicine in the last decade. Unfortunately, most of the contributors to the F & S survey represent large plants or companies, so that comparisons in the small plant categories were not possible.

This study represents a general view of the status of occupational medicine within industry. It would be necessary to conduct individual studies within major industrial segments, such as manufacturing, construction, mining, and public utilities, to produce more detailed information regarding the status of occupational medicine. We hope to accomplish this over the next few years.

1
The Political Background: A Legislative History of OSHA

The founding of a federal agency to safeguard the health and safety of American workers on the job grew out of a new awareness of the magnitude of health and safety hazards present in the workplace and an apparent commitment by the government to limit those dangers. The Occupational Safety and Health Administration (OSHA), as the federal agency was called, was spawned amidst considerable controversy, because its creation and subsequent activities, despite its seemingly non-controversial mandate to protect worker health and safety, raised two issues that were simultaneously economic and political: cost and control.

The standards approved by OSHA for maintaining a modicum of safety and preventing work-induced illness or disease required that firms revamp their operations; the changes were grouped under the heading of environmental controls. New mechanical features were to be introduced into plants to assure that noxious fumes, harmful concentrations of toxic materials, excessive noise, or lethal machinery did not damage the health nor endanger the safety of those who worked in the plants. Controls of this sort required allocation of company funds, and many companies objected to this use of their resources, largely because they did not wish to absorb the cost. Objections to cost shaded into hostility toward any and all efforts that forced companies to cede control over parts of their operations. In this light, any program designed to monitor company compliance with federal regulations or to require redesign of plant facilities to meet minimum health and safety specifications represented an infringement upon managerial prerogatives. From the perspective of OSHA's most ardent supporters, public interest groups led by Ralph Nader and many labor unions, however, that was just the point. The introduction of national legislation to protect the health and safety of workers served as the means to redress the at best uneven record of firms in protecting their workers. Outside supervision of firms' activities to protect worker health and safety afforded workers new or additional protection; the redesign of plant facilities eliminated reliance upon protective measures that were solely discretionary.

Since its inception, then, OSHA has been buffeted by opposing forces. The battle lines have been formed around a series of questions about cost and control: who pays; who is responsible; what is required to protect workers; and who decides what is required?

BACKGROUND

Industrial processes have long posed hazards of health and safety to the workers who were engaged in them. In both the production of textiles and the mining of coal, two of the world's oldest industries, laborers faced the strong possibility of receiving incapacitating injuries at work or contracting chronic and debilitating illnesses. Close contact with chemicals and poisons made the bleaching and dyeing of cotton or flax fabrics a dangerous occupation; extended labor in subterranean mine seams made miners vulnerable to the collapse of shafts and the combustion of methane gas present in the coal dust. One vivid image of the health hazards of manufacturing has been conveyed by the term "mad hatter": the neurological damage to the makers of hats, brought on by the use of mercury in their manufacture, gave rise to the seemingly aberrant behavior of the hatters.

At times, industrial innovation, while increasing the productive capacity of the regional or national economy, has also exacerbated the threat to the health and safety of workers. The first mechanized handlooms, for example, placed a massive strain on the eyes of children who worked them, and early blindness was a common result. The Davy safety lamp, which was introduced into English and American mines in the early 19th century, reduced the immediate likelihood of methane explosions, but encouraged the mining industry to have shafts dug deeper, which led to more deaths from cave-ins and underground explosions.

The industrial development of the United States after World War II was marked by the introduction of a vast number of new manufacturing techniques. These processes relied heavily upon metals, chemicals, and petrochemical derivatives to facilitate the production of new materials or to form intermediate products from which final goods were made. For example, beryllium was used in the manufacture of cathode tubes for television; cobalt and cadmium in the manufacture of airplanes. In the agricultural sector, pesticides and chemical fertilizers came into common use. Plastics, first developed on a wide scale as petrochemical derivatives in the 1930s, were used to preserve perishable foods, to contain products of all sorts, and for clothing. Moreover, these chemical derivatives began to play an important role in intermediate industrial processes: vinyl chloride, for example, formed the polymer chain polyvinyl chloride, which was used in the manufacture of a large number of household and industrial items. Finally, radioactive materials were created and stored for use in industry, medicine, and war.

The prosperity of the 1960s raised expectations that the injuries and afflictions that accompanied industrial and agricultural labor no longer need plague the workforce of the United States. Up until the 1960s the regulation of health and safety matters had fallen primarily to the states and private agencies, which often operated in an uneven and desultory fashion. The major protection afforded workers came only after injuries had been sustained: since the early 1900s state workmen's compensation laws had served as the means through which companies and individuals settled claims for injuries incurred on the job. Private agencies, in particular the American National Standards Institute (ANSI), had established standards for protection of worker health and safety that had the approval of the industries involved. It was ANSI, for example, that set the standard governing what injuries had to be reported to state agencies. Known as Z16, this rule required the reporting of any injry which so harmed the individual that he was unable to return to work for a full day after the injury was incurred. These standards formed the main body of preventive measures to protect workers.

The federal government did have some authority over health and safety matters through the Walsh-Healey Act of 1936, which gave the government the right to apply health and safety standards to workplaces of firms doing more than $10,000 worth of business with the government.

By the late 1960s a growing awareness of the environmental dangers posed to the health of the population in general was coupled with the heightened expectation of the possibility of political and social change and led to the first significant attempts to make workplace protection a national policy. At the same time the extent of health and safety risks in the workplace was emphasized in several ways. While mining disasters, such as the explosion in Farmington, West Virginia, in 1968 that claimed 86 lives, as well as mounting evidence of the disabling and deadly effects of breathing coal dust over a lifetime in the mines, received nationwide attention, studies of the effects of other chemicals upon the long-term health of exposed workers, pioneered in the United States by Dr. Irving Selikoff, led to the conclusion that exposure to certain toxic substances increased the risk of developing cancer. These latter studies encouraged epidemiological investigation of the relationship between work environment and cancer.

LEGISLATION

In an address on the nation's manpower needs in 1968, Lyndon Johnson enunciated the principle that protection of worker health and safety was in the national interest. The drive to develop a national occupational safety and health act had entered its first stage. Johnson's withdrawal from the presidential race later that year deprived the movement of presidential impetus. Instead, the issue of occupational health and safety received extensive congressional consideration in the first years of the Nixon presidency. In 1969 support for national legislation was drawn from two main sources: public interest groups, led by Ralph Nader, and labor unions, but especially the Oil, Chemical, and Atomic Workers Union and, to a lesser degree, the United Automobile Workers. Although business interests opposed any legislation on occupational health and safety in 1968, the next year they rallied behind a proposal put forth by Representative William Steiger of Wisconsin. Steiger's bill established a tripartite authority to set standards, enforce their maintenance, and review appeals. The Steiger proposal emphasized the voluntary aspects of enforcement; the authority vested in the Department of Labor to set standards permitted the official in charge of occupational safety and health to use his discretion in pursuing charges of violations. By contrast, a proposal launched by Nader's public interest group and the AFL-CIO made enforcement standards obligatory; moreover, it vested the setting and enforcement of standards within one body, the Department of Labor. The bill that grew out of this proposal was promoted by Representative Daniels of Pennsylvania and Senator Harrison Williams from New Jersey.[1]

In the end, a compromise, the Williams-Steiger bill, was adopted. The Occupational Safety and Health Act of 1970 approved by President Nixon set forth the principle that all workers should be afforded protection from injury or health hazards. With that claim as its point of departure, the act set the framework for the adoption—or creation—of standards whereby the health and safety of workers in the workplace would be assured. It fell to OSHA, a bureau established in the Department of Labor, to set standards, for which the act provided three different means. Standards set by private agencies were incorporated into OSHA's body of standards. In addition to those established by ANSI, threshold level values of toxic substances found in the workplace (designated by a daily maximum of parts per million in the atmosphere) and approved by the American Committee of Government and Industrial Hygienists (ACGIH), another quasi-private agency, were taken up by OSHA. The act also provided for the testing of permanent standards for toxic substances, but as OSHA's first years revealed, the adoption of these new standards proved to be laborious. (The first to enter OSHA's list was asbestos, which was listed in 1972.) While permanent standards for allowable levels of toxicity were under study, OSHA had scope to adopt emergency standards in the interim, but not for periods longer than six months.

The Occupational Safety and Health Act placed responsibility for the enforcement of these standards in the Department of Labor as well. OSHA was empowered to enforce standards by sending out inspectors to sites, citing violations, and imposing fines. Workers were able to initiate action by contacting OSHA; violations cited were to be posted at the workplace. Gradually OSHA

---

[1] For a history of the legislative battles, see Joseph A. Page and Mary-Win O'Brien, *Bitter Wages* (New York: Grossman Publishers, 1973).

acquired a staff of nearly 1500 inspectors for all the workplaces that came within the purview of the act. As part of the compromise embodied in the Williams-Steiger bill, review of OSHA's actions and appeals were handled by an independent commission appointed by the president.

The Occupational Safety and Health Act also set forth the necessity of encouraging government research into the toxicity of substances found in the workplace and of training employers and employees to recognize health and safety hazards. The act created the National Institute of Occupational Safety and Health (NIOSH) as the research division empowered to conduct studies of toxic substances, which were to form the basis upon which OSHA would adopt new permanent standards of health hazards. Although not specified in the original act, the Nixon administration chose to transform the Bureau of Occupational Safety and Health (BOSH), a minor office in the Department of Health, Education, and Welfare, into NIOSH. Its headquarters remained in Cincinnati; after 1975 it was subordinated to the Center for Disease Control (CDC) based in Atlanta.

The Nixon administration's attitude toward the program of workplace health and safety regulation was at best mixed: though the administration had supported the passage of legislation creating such an agency, albeit a weaker version than the one finally approved by Congress, its policies in the first years of the program damaged the effectiveness of OSHA as a regulatory entity. Slow to appoint a full complement of inspectors, the Nixon administration contributed to the muddying of OSHA's ability to set standards by adopting—in short order— the consensus standards developed by ANSI and ACGIH. The act had allowed for the agency to take time to develop a much shorter list of standards, which would improve the efficacy of the overall program and at the same time be less confusing to those to whom the program applied. In addition, in its sensitivity to underlying business opposition to OSHA, the Nixon administration, through OSHA's first head, Arthur Guenther, hinted at easing enforcement of OSHA standards in 1972 in return for campaign contributions to the Nixon reelection effort.

ENFORCEMENT EFFORTS

During the Nixon era OSHA was plagued by weak or misdirected enforcement: minor, that is, technical, safety violations would be cited, while major health and safety hazards were ignored. The limited number of inspectors reduced the likelihood that a plant would face inspection in the short run, and attempts to monitor farmwork, where the workforce was largely non-organized and migrant in character, proved especially difficult. According to OSHA policy, employers were to be notified of conditions in need of correction after violations were found, then given a grace period to make the requisite corrections before fines were imposed. On average, OSHA fines amounted to less than $50 per violation during the first half-decade of the agency's existence.[2]

For all that, OSHA did set about its task of determining safe levels of toxic substances. With the assistance of NIOSH, it slowly developed a list of materials whose ingestion appeared to increase the risk of developing cancer over the long term. In 1972 the agency set a permanent standard for asbestos; the next year it adopted a threshold limit for a group of 14 substances known to cause cancer. Vinyl chloride was placed on the list in 1974 and coke oven emissions were listed in 1976. Then in 1978 a standard was set for exposure to benzene. The inclusion of these substances on a list of permanent standards and the limits of tolerable exposure were subjects of political disputation. By and large, efforts to incorporate these chemicals on the list were spearheaded by groups outside of OSHA, namely, public interest groups and labor unions like the Oil, Chemical, and Atomic Workers Union or the United Rubberworkers. Moreover, the threshold levels did not go unchallenged: industry spokespeople tended to argue for thresholds higher than those finally approved; public interest and union spokespeople tended to militate for threshold levels below those set.

Arguments of this sort represented one form of the debate that continued to take place about OSHA's role and effectiveness. Initially, an awakening to environmental concerns had transformed the attitude of the American public at large about the hazards that existed in the workplace, and labor unions—in varying degrees—became increasingly responsive to demands about protecting worker health and safety. In fact, the specter of environmental poisoning helped fuel concern that OSHA's attempt to limit worker susceptibility to serious health hazards represented merely a rearguard effort. Businesses tended to accept only grudgingly the need to regulate the environment of the workplace. From that corner, opposition to OSHA took shape primarily in a campaign to restrict the scope of OSHA's operations. In 1972 Senator Carl Curtis of Nebraska introduced a proposal to deny OSHA authority to inspect and fine small businesses, those that employed less than 25 workers. Curtis based his argument on the financial hardship imposed on these businesses to modify their plants to conform to OSHA standards. Supporters of OSHA's broad coverage of firms countered by noting that small firms oftentimes posed greater health and safety hazards to their workers than larger ones.

By the mid-1970s the debate about OSHA policy had shifted to the principles upon which the agency had been founded. OSHA's reliance upon standards that established acceptable safety practices and tolerable concentrations of toxic materials in the workplace was predicated upon the past practice of other quasi-regulatory bodies. Private agencies like ANSI had resorted to the use of standards, and the federal government had applied a system of standards to guaran-

---

[2] Les Boden and David Wegman, "Increasing OSHA's Clout: Sixty Million New Inspectors," *Working Papers for a New Society*, May–June 1978.

tee the health and safety of workers covered by the Walsh-Healey Act. This reliance upon standards also implied recognition of the importance of controlling the environment of the workplace as the prerequisite to limiting exposure of workers to health and safety hazards. If the number of units of a toxic substance present in the atmosphere of the workplace were to be limited to a given amount, then workers would have some assurance that they had not been unduly exposed and threatened with later illness or death. Similarly, if the workplace were to be designed to eliminate certain safety risks or certain work rules were to be invoked to minimize the danger of accidents to workers, then workers once again would be assured of a modicum of safety on the job.

In both cases the protection afforded the workers was preventive and probabilistic. Substances that might endanger their health were removed from the scene; unsafe conditions were similarly eliminated. Neither move attempted to calculate *ex post* the effect on worker safety or health. For long-term exposure to toxic substances and carcinogens, there was no alternative: a whole generation of workers would have been ravaged by the time the disease appeared. This is hardly a theoretical point: an estimated 8 to 9 million individuals were exposed to asbestos before the dangers of asbestosis were known and publicized at large; chronic illness or death may afflict hundreds of thousands of those exposed over a 30-year period. Standards suggest what courses of action ought to be undertaken to reduce or eliminate the likely harm to health or injury posed by the presence of unsafe conditions or noxious substances.

OPPOSITION TO OSHA

Critics of OSHA, mainly but not exclusively from the right, attacked the need for pre-set standards by challenging the program's effectiveness in preventing deaths, injuries, and illnesses. When OSHA was formed in 1970, an estimated 14,000 individuals lost their lives each year in job-related accidents or health hazards; roughly 2,000,000 were injured or disabled as a result of mishaps on the job. The first studies of the number of injuries incurred at work after OSHA came into existence indicated a small reduction in the number of job-related injuries. The most definitive study, conducted by John Mendeloff, measured changes in the number of job-related injuries in California after 1970 and indicated a 2 to 5 percent drop in the number.[3]

On the right, critics argued for an indirect system of controls that measured the effectiveness of regulations and/or incentives solely on the basis of the number of injuries or deaths prevented: in short, a method based on a retrospective

---

[3] John Mendeloff, "An Evaluation of the OSHA Program's Effect on Workplace Injury Rates: Evidence from California, 1974" (Office of the Assistant Secretary for Policy, Evaluation, and Research, U.S. Department of Labor, 1976). Also *Regulating Safety* (Cambridge, Mass.: MIT Press, 1979).

count. Robert Smith, writing in 1976 under the auspices of the American Enterprise Institute, proposed a new method known as the injury tax. According to Smith and other academic proponents of the tax,[4] the prevention of occupational health and safety problems would be left to a system determined by economic incentives for employers. Advocates of the plan argued that employers would be free to choose whatever method they wished to control workplace injuries or illnesses, as long as they were prepared to pay a fee or tax for the harm done to their employees.

The criticism of OSHA from the right was rooted in neo-classical economic theory. As such, it represented the first major effort to make cost the point of departure in considerations of occupational health and safety, and hinted as well at the broader role cost-benefit analysis would be accorded. In terms of an injury tax, for example, the employer was given sole responsibility for determining the relative value of the tax assessed against him for health problems encountered by his employees as opposed to the cost of improving work conditions to safeguard his employees' health and safety. At this stage employee input or knowledge of the conditions under which he labored was cast aside: the firm determined the method by which the workers' health and safety would be protected. Thus the injury tax proved appealing to businesses that wished to assert all managerial prerogatives.

On the other hand, opposition to the introduction of economic incentives and cost-benefit analysis in health and safety matters grew out of concern that worker health and safety would be jeopardized as a result. Notions like an injury tax would transform occupational health and safety into a matter to be weighed by an employer and his accountant. The record of adherence to the reporting of accidents would be available only in the relevant tax forms. More generally, the reporting of injuries and other threats to health would be invisible to those who were affected.[5] When OSHA was founded, both employers and employees were given rights and responsibilities to assure a safe working environment; under cost-benefit analysis worker safety and health once again became the province of management rights. In fact, it was possible to see a disproportionate share of the responsibility fall upon the shoulders of employees, who might be deemed more susceptible to health and safety risks and find themselves excluded from employment.

Under cost-benefit analysis, the benefit of preventing illness, injury, and death to workers was set against the cost of providing the benefit. A social cost was affixed to the injuries, illnesses, and deaths that would occur, or, alternatively, methods of reducing the number of mishaps at work would be compared

---

[4] Robert Stewart Smith, *The Occupational Safety and Health Act* (Washington, D.C.: American Enterprise Institute, 1976); Albert L. Nichols and Richard Zeckhauser, "Government Comes to the Workplace: An Assessment of OSHA," *Public Interest*, Fall 1977.

[5] See Boden and Wegman, *supra*.

on a dollar-for-dollar basis. Advocates of cost-benefit analysis like Murray Weidenbaum, who later became chief of the Council of Economic Advisors in the Reagan administration, argued that its basis was utilitarian in nature: how best to reduce a specified number of illnesses, injuries, or deaths for a given amount of dollars allocated to that end. As an economic argument drawn from microeconomic tenets, the cost-benefit method did not appear to draw distinctions among ways in which occupational mishaps and diseases would be reduced, although, in keeping with the method's theoretical underpinning, it was always assumed that the firm, rather than the workers, would determine the way to proceed. Proponents suggested that the method provided a means by which the costs of assuring occupational health and safety could be controlled by the firms involved.

Opponents responded with a moral and an economic argument.[6] On the one hand, they argued that the introduction of cost-benefit analysis into occupational health and safety matters represented a kind of triage, whereby, for a given amount of funds allocated for the purpose, some employees would be allowed to suffer injury, illness, or death. On the other hand, they raised the question of social cost, that is, the cost to society of actions taken by the firm. The size of the fine assessed—under the injury tax plan—would have a crucial effect upon the employer's response to health and safety needs in his plant. If the tax were set at a high enough figure, the firm would be obliged to maintain quite strict standards of health and safety. Special consideration also had to be given to the time period over which cost and benefit were calculated, especially for work-induced diseases. Under these circumstances, resort to cost-benefit analysis might not prove as alluring as those advocating lowering costs had originally thought. And cost, rather than maintenance of health and safety in the workplace, was the central concern of the advocates of cost-benefit analysis.

Although cost-benefit analysis represented a new development in the theoretical debate about the direction of OSHA, it did not differ markedly in practical terms from other methods of limiting costs that businesses had pressed for since OSHA's inception. These called for minimizing costs in pursuit of the goal of reducing the number of work-related injuries and deaths. Advocates argued for reliance upon protective devices, for which the workers themselves were responsible, rather than engineering controls: ear plugs or ear muffs could be used to ward off excessive noises in the workplace; oral respirators would prevent ingestion of toxic materials in the factory or on the farm. If workers did not avail themselves of these protective devices, they would then be seen as responsible for damaging their own health.

---

[6] Mendeloff, in *Regulating Safety, supra*, distinguishes between economic and moral (or legal) claims about occupational health and safety. More recently, Steven Kelman, who wrote *Regulating America, Regulating Sweden* (Cambridge, Mass.: MIT Press, 1981), has argued that economic evaluations of occupational health and safety ignore the human-rights notion embodied in the principle of protecting worker health and safety.

In turn, critics of reliance upon protective devices argued that workers did not create the work environment in which they toiled and that such voluntary measures oftentimes would simply fail to protect the health of those affected.[7] The exposure of workers in a pesticide-making plant in Hopewell, Virginia, to chlordecone, in 1975 represented a prime example of the dangers of relying upon voluntary protective measures. These critics charged that knowledge of the dangers of exposure was required before workers could assume any responsibility for protecting themselves; moreover, environmental controls eliminated any possibility that voluntary actions would be shirked by either employer or employee.

OSHA's operations were also challenged from the left.[8] While these critics did not dispute the reasonableness of the goals of the program, in contrast to those on the right who felt that the costs did not justify the results, they expressed doubts about the methods used to achieve these goals and about the effectiveness of OSHA as an administrative agency. Their criticism was founded on the notion that violations of health and safety standards were commonplace; in addition, both voluntary compliance and the efforts undertaken by OSHA were insufficient to meet the demands of maintaining health and safety conditions.

In particular, Boden and Wegman pointed to the limitations of enforcing health and safety conditions through teams of inspectors available to the agency. Instead, they argued for greater activism on the local level. Drawing from the model of the organization of occupational health and safety monitoring in Sweden, they contended that the federal government should encourage, through training programs, the local union members—for non-union plants a somewhat more problematic undertaking—to gain a detailed knowledge of health and safety matters in the plant and serve as safety inspectors, akin to the union shop stewards. As employees in their own workplaces, these inspectors would have strong incentives to assure that the work environment was safe and free from health hazards. The scope of such a program far exceeded OSHA's provision for training workers and represented a direct effort to link improvements in working conditions with a transformation of rights and responsibilities in the workplace. For the time being, the proposal has not been implemented.

One further element was introduced into the worker health and safety calculus in the late 1970s. The new consciousness of the omnipresence of health and safety hazards had given rise, by the early 1970s, to a new emphasis upon preventive techniques to reduce risks. The engineering controls stipulated by OSHA's standards, in fact, represented one version of preventive protection for workers. Another version, though, also took shape during this period: preventive

---

[7] See, for example, Samuel S. Epstein, *The Politics of Cancer* (San Francisco: Sierra Club Books, 1978).

[8] See Boden and Wegman, *supra*.

medicine. Based on the common-sense notion that health hazards could more readily be treated by their elimination beforehand rather than after the fact, preventive medical practices were encouraged. Although these practices appeared to complement efforts to diminish risks to health in the workplace through environmental controls, they also redirected the focus of occupational health policy back to the individual. Two difficulties presented themselves: individual workers might be deemed more susceptible to health hazards and not be hired or individuals might be held responsible for what befell them.

COURT RULINGS

As the 1970s drew to a close, the applicability of cost-benefit analysis in health and safety matters and the responsibility of the individual in preventing health risks on the job came under judicial review. Those who wished to diminish OSHA's role sought relief in court on the basis of costs involved; they argued that the government should be obliged to apply least-cost or cost-benefit analysis methods to the protection of worker health and safety. Supporters of OSHA also brought suit, seeking to sustain OSHA's guiding principle of preserving the health and safety of Americans at the workplace without regard to cost. The legislation itself had provided that the establishment of standards take into account the "feasibility" of reaching and maintaining standards. The act also made reference to the financial demands placed on small businesses covered by OSHA, and special assistance was to be provided for these businesses to enable them to comply with the act. In general, however, the issue of cost was relegated to secondary status. (In the debate about creating OSHA the economic arguments raised centered on the overall loss of productivity as a result of man-hours lost because of illness or injury.)

The first of the two cases to make its way through the courts concerned the damage wrought by byssinosis, or brown-lung disease, a debilitating—and ultimately fatal—disease in which those affected develop a condition akin to emphysema and bronchial asthma. Textile workers had unusually high rates of the disease, and it had been identified in the early 1970s as a consequence of ingesting cotton or flax dust, particles of which pervaded the atmosphere of textile plants in the South. In a correlative case, a textile worker who had contracted brown-lung disease and had been a heavy smoker of cigarettes sought damages from the company in which he worked.

By the time the test case on the applicability of cost-benefit analysis had reached the United States Supreme Court, the Reagan administration had come to power. During the 1970s Reagan had suggested that OSHA be disbanded or, at the least, that matters of occupational health and safety be determined on the basis of an analysis of the value of the benefit provided against the cost of providing it. The direction of both public and private programs of occupational health hung in the balance. If the Supreme Court were to rule in favor of the linkage between costs and benefits, occupational health and safety measures would become more voluntarist in nature and most likely would be substantially curtailed. If the Supreme Court were to rule that cost-benefit analysis was inapplicable under the circumstances, then the overall direction of health and safety policy devised in the 1970s would be maintained, although the Reagan administration, much like the Nixon administration, would still have significant leeway within its purview to weaken OSHA's effectiveness. In March 1981 the Court reached its decision: cost-benefit analysis could not be used to determine what health and safety measures would be undertaken to comply with OSHA's mandate.

The Supreme Court's decision on the second test case, however, muddied the issue somewhat. Because the Court did not find that exposure to benzene posed a high risk, it ruled that the standard used to protect workers exposed to the petrochemical was not valid. OSHA's mandate remained intact, but proof of high risk posed new difficulties in its implementation.

2
Environmental Factors in Occupationally Induced Diseases

The work environment contains hundreds of known health hazards and many suspected and potentially dangerous ones. Such hazards as they relate to the workers' health can be placed in three distinct categories: chemical substances, biological substances, and physical agents. These hazards can be toxic, carcinogens or mutagens, teratogens, or irritants.

CHEMICAL HAZARDS

Chemical substances represent the most widespread and serious workplace hazards. Such substances can enter the body via inhalation, skin contact, or ingestion.

Inhalation is the most common route of entry. Inhaled agents are gases, vapors, fumes, and dust, substances that are omnipresent in the air in the manufacturing industries. Some substances can kill instantly, but the majority cause chronic irritation or delayed organ damage. Also, inhaled substances can be carcinogens or mutagens or teratogens. Hazardous agents introduced into the body via the airways include:

inert gases, such as carbon monoxide and hydrogen sulfide, that can cause asphyxiation,

soluble gases, such as sulfur dioxide and ammonia, that cause inflammation of the upper respiratory tract. Other gases, such as chlorine, nitrogen dioxide, phosgene, and ozone, attack the lower respiratory tract and can cause permanent lung disease,

gases of low water solubility, such as volatile liquids that generally pass through the alveoli, enter the bloodstream, and cause selective organ damage, and
dusts and fumes that are often harmless but sometimes cause respiratory and lung disorders, such as airway irritation or obstruction, fibrosis, or emphysema.

Workers can be protected from inhaling hazardous agents through the installation of engineering controls and use of protective equipment. Although disliked by the workers, protective equipment like respirators is becoming more and more prevalent in manufacturing plants where inhalation of dangerous substances is a real concern. New engineering controls and improved ventilation systems also reduce dusts and fumes.

It is more difficult to protect workers against hazardous agents that enter the body through the skin. Most substances cannot penetrate the skin due to a natural protective barrier, but many agents react with the skin to cause "industrial dermatitis," a very common occurrence in the manufacturing industries. Some, however, penetrate the (intact or broken) skin and enter the bloodstream. Agents penetrating the skin can cause selective organ damage and even cancer.

Occupational hazards from ingestion of harmful agents are the least likely. In most plants, eating, smoking, and drinking are not permitted in the production area. Workers rather have a well-segregated eating area and are urged to change out of their workclothes and to wash before eating.

Disease-Producing Actions of Chemical Substances

Chemical substances can cause damage by various mechanisms, that is, physical, chemical, and physiological.

Agents Causing Physical Damage. Many hazardous agents physically assault organ systems by removing surface lipids, denaturation, or other skin carrier damage. Physical injury causes skin irritation, cellular damage, and even necrosis. Effects range from eye and skin irritation to respiratory tract inflammation and edema, and to gastrointestinal tract effects, such as nausea, vomiting, and diarrhea. Agents causing physical damage include: liquids with a solvent or emulsifying action, acid or alkaline soluble gases, vapors, particulates, and inert gases. High concentrations of inert gases can cause death by asphyxiation due to simple oxygen displacement.

The control of hazardous agents that assault the body by physical mechanisms is rather simple. Appropriate clothes, protective equipment, and local medications help to minimize exposure. Environmental controls regarding emissions of particulates or other irritants in the workplace also eliminate the danger posed by inhalants. Finally, if exposure occurs, most effects are transient and easily handled by first aid procedures. Unless there is persistent exposure and lack of hygiene and first aid, the long-term effects of injury posed by the physical action of chemical agents are negligible. Of course accidental exposure to high concentrations of inert gases can be fatal, but this event would result from a safety rather than a medical problem.

Toxic Substances (Agents Causing Chemical Damage). Hazardous agents in this category disrupt normal chemical processes by combining with chemicals in the body to form substances that are either highly toxic or that cannot perform their original function.

Toxicity is inherent in many chemical substances and careful hygiene and safety procedures are necessary to insure proper employee protection. There are several types of mechanisms of chemical toxicity. Some chemical agents disrupt the production and balance of electrolytes, with an imbalance of the acids and bases resulting in acidosis or alkalosis. By directly combining with body compounds, chemical toxins destroy or alter the function of the body constituent. For instance, by combining with hemoglobin, carbon monoxide replaces oxygen and causes anoxia and eventually death.

Sometimes external chemical agents cause the body to produce excessive amounts of normal substances, such as in the case of allergic reactions when an abnormal amount of histamine is released due to exposure to a chemical stimulant. Chelation is another way of disrupting body function. In chelation, an external agent produces a new compound by binding, and thus removing the metals found in cells. More commonly, however, chelating agents are used to remove toxic substances from the body, such as in lead or mercury poisoning.

Preventing toxicity from chemically acting agents is much more difficult than from those that have physical effects. Damage can be serious before symptoms become obvious. Health monitoring is very important in this area and it must be performed using more sophisticated techniques than those necessary with physically acting substances. Still, chemically induced toxicity is relatively easy to prevent by adhering to strict hygiene procedures and by some health monitoring.

Agents Causing Physiological Disorders. This type of chemical hazard is the most serious, as it is not well understood and often long latent periods occur before the effects become symptomatic, at which point the outcome is often catastrophic. The presence and importance of physiologically hazardous agents are primarily responsible for the creation and widespread applicability of employee health monitoring.

Physiological effects are primarily caused by the abnormal function of enzyme systems. Most agents have an affinity for certain enzyme systems and therefore affect those systems exclusively or almost so.

BIOLOGICAL HAZARDS

Biological hazards include insects and mites, molds, yeasts, fungi, bacteria, and viruses, which cause infectious diseases, parasitism, and toxic and allergic reactions. Occupations most often exposed to pathogenic microorganisms include farmers, veterinarians, meat process workers, rendering and tanning workers, bakers, cattle breeders, construction workers, cooks, health workers.

Occupationally induced infectious diseases are usually caused by viruses carried by animals and zoonoses, such as anthrax and psittacosis. Bacteria enter the body through minor skin cuts and abrasions but occasionally bacteria can also be inhaled. Fungal disease, although rare, sometimes occurs in agricultural workers and others employed in outdoor jobs.

Workers exposed to plant matter may also develop local and systemic reactions, ranging from dermatitis to asthma and allergies. Herbicide and pesticide residue on plants and fruits may also prove toxic to those handling them.

Common infections, such as respiratory problems, including tuberculosis, can also be considered as occupationally induced if contracted by a worker while performing the duties of his office. Particularly vulnerable are hospital and laboratory workers. Tuberculosis tests are routinely given to prospective hospital employees and also are part of periodic physical examinations.

In summary, disorders caused by biological hazards include animal-carried diseases, such as brucellosis, psittacosis, anthrax, tularemia, erysipeloid, Q fever, equine encephalomyelitis, mite dermatitis, and those caused by agents present in water, air, or soil, such as histoplasmosis, coccidioidomycosis, blastomycosis, larva migrans, tetanus, leptospirosis and schistosomiasis.

The best prevention is proper worker immunization if a vaccine exists. Otherwise, early diagnosis is also important and company physicians are encouraged to educate the workers to recognize the symptoms of certain diseases.

PHYSICAL HAZARDS

Physical hazards, such as noise, heat, radiation, pressure, and vibration, can also cause serious health problems if exposure is prolonged and an evaluation of health status is not performed regularly.

Noise

Noise is omnipresent in the work environment and auditory problems are the single most prevalent complaints of industrial workers. Nealry 40 percent of all workers in the United States are exposed to noise levels that can cause hearing problems. Exposure to high noise levels for prolonged periods of time may cause hearing loss, which can be temporary or permanent.

Hearing loss can be prevented through the use of protective equipment or engineering controls. Often workers disregard voluntary prophylactic methods that they find an annoyance. Most occupational medicine programs in industries where workers are exposed to high noise levels regularly assess hearing acuity.

Noisy environments contribute to vocal cord dysfunction resulting from straining the vocal cords in order to be heard over the din. Such dysfunctions include cord nodules, polyps, or chronic laryngitis. Other environmental factors, such as dust, smoke, and fumes, also aggravate this condition.

Radiation

There are two main types of radiation, ionizing and nonionizing. The deleterious effects of high and moderate doses, or ionizing, radiation have been well documented and are not disputed by anyone. However, the effects of low-level, or nonionizing, radiation have not been analyzed sufficiently and are now believed to be much more harmful than previously suspected. The proliferation of nuclear plants, the extensive testing of nuclear weapons on the United States mainland in the 1950s, and the frequent exposure of patients to medical procedures involving low-dose radiation have brought the issue into focus.

A study conducted by Dr. Thomas Najarian[41] on former workers of the Portsmouth Naval Shipyard showed that cancer deaths were significantly higher among nuclear workers than the general population. Leukemia deaths were five times higher. Similar results were observed among army personnel involved in nuclear weapons testing and in studies of populations that lived in the path of fallout clouds resulting from nuclear weapons tests. However, the methods of data collection and the statistical methods employed are controversial and there is no clear-cut evidence relating cancer incidence with low-dose radiation.

It is also theorized that low-dose radiation might become carcinogenic if present with other potentially carcinogenic substances. Also, radiation exposure, even at low doses may cause mutagenicity.

Employees exposed to low-dose radiation are those working in such facilities as nuclear power plants, nuclear weapons plants and testing sites, nuclear submarines, radar facilities, nuclear fuel manufacturing plants, medical products plants (x-ray, heart pacemakers), testing laboratories.

Ionizing radiation includes: x-rays, gamma-rays (photons), beta particles (electrons), alpha particles, neutrons, and other nuclear components. The largest source of ionizing radiation exposure is from medical and dental x-ray units. Such exposure presents an occupational hazard to medical personnel.

Another large source of x-ray exposure is represented by nondestructive testing and analytical instruments used in research laboratories. Other sources of ionizing radiation include neutron activation equipment, instruments using sealed radioactive sources (cobalt-60, cesium-137, indium-192), thickness gauges, luminous signs, flow measuring devices.

The acute effects of ionizing radiation exposure vary depending on the organ at risk and the dose schedule. Common effects include sterility, pulmonary fibrosis, nephritis and hypertension, brain and spinal cord necrosis, atrophy. However, the most serious effects of radiation exposure is carcinogenicity, with latent periods of 20 years or more, and mutagenicity that might not be evident for several generations.

Electromagnetic radiation produces changes in biological systems either via photochemical (ultraviolet) or thermal modes (infrared, microwave). Table 1 lists the various types of electromagnetic radiation and their health effects.

Generally, nonionizing radiation is not found to be harmful, except in selected cases where accidental exposure causes serious trauma. There has been some speculation, however, that microwave radiation could affect the central nervous system (CNS) and induce reproductive disorders. Microwaves are currently generated by hundreds of electrical sources from radar installations to television and household appliances, which has prompted some to call the United States a giant microwave oven.

Potential damage from microwave radiation became a national issue when it was revealed that the Russians were bombarding the United States embassy in

Table 1: Health Effects of Nonionizing Radiation

Type of Radiation	Wavelength	Biological and Health Effects
Ultraviolet	100-400 nm	Erythema Skin cancer Photosensitization Keratoconjunctivitis Corneal epithelium damage
Infrared	750-10^6 nm	Skin burns Whole body heating
Lasers		Protein denaturation Retinal burns Macular damage and eye loss Skin burns
Radiofrequency	10^6 nm-10 MHz	
Microwave	10 MHz-300 GHz	Burns Central nervous system effects? Reproductive ? Ocular cataracts

Moscow with microwaves used as an elaborate bugging and jamming system. Investigators claim that the incidence of cancer and the number of birth defects was higher among embassy personnel. Other professionals exposed to large amounts of microwave radiation, such as air traffic controllers and radar operators, also claim increased disability due to this exposure. However, other studies, one recently performed by the National Academy of Sciences, show no ill effects from microwave radiation among exposed individuals. Undoubtedly the microwave danger issue will continue to be debated.

Pressure, Temperature, and Vibration

Extremes in pressure occur in construction (tunnels), in diving, and in high altitude flying. Almost always a physician monitors workers' health in such operations on a continuing basis.

Temperature extremes occur in many manufacturing processes. High temperatures occur in metal working operations. Extreme cold environments are found in meat-packing plants, in deep-freeze food production, and storage operations. Acclimatization is better in hot than cold environments. Workers exposed to low temperatures over long periods may show a high incidence of chronic muscle and joint pains and upper respiratory tract problems. On the other hand, the effects of a hot environment, such as an increase in body temperature and pulse rate, are readily reversible. More serious complications of exposure to high temperatures include: heat cramps, exhaustion, or heat stroke. One of the most serious problems associated with long-term exposure to cold temperatures is hypothermia, which is often fatal, caused by vasodilation and rapid body heat loss.

Exposure to vibration affects nearly one million workers in the construction, farming, and trucking industries. Prolonged exposure to vibration causes joint deformations, gastrointestinal problems, loss of visual acuity, and interferes with normal sleeping and eating habits.

GENETIC PREDISPOSITION

One of the most elusive aspects of pre-employment evaluations is the genetic risk factor in occupationally induced disease. It is estimated that 12 million Americans carry true genetic disease, the manifestation of which can be greatly influenced by the individual's environment.

A recent report of a confirmed inherited chromosome aberration within a family associated with cancer of the kidney further demonstrates that risk of cancer is not borne equally by all, and that exposure of genetically predisposed individuals to specific hazardous environments might trigger the early appearance of cancer.

A few cancers appear to be inherited with a pattern of dominant inheritance, such as retinoblastoma and adenocarcinomatosis; others show an increased risk, such as breast cancer. A careful pre-employment examination, including a complete family health history, should identify individuals at risk.

The identification of individuals with genetic markers that would eventually lead to malignancies remains problematic as a prevention method. One group of markers that signify genetic predisposition or susceptibility to certain diseases are the human leukocyte antigens (HLA). To date, scientists have identified more than 40 diseases that can be related to the HLA profile of the patient. Currently, the most striking correlation between HLA and disease can be found in ankylosing spondylitis, but other immune disorders may be involved, such as Hodgkin's disease and leukemia. It is premature to predict that genetic markers might have a predictive role in occupational medicine. In ankylosing spondylitis, for instance, almost all males with the disease have HLA type B27, whereas any male with B27 has a 20 percent chance of developing the disease.

PSYCHOLOGICAL AND MENTAL PROBLEMS

Large corporations have addressed the problem of employee mental health in a similar fashion as they have met his physical health requirements. Work stress, aggravated by family and social problems or poor physical health often render the employee incapable of performing his job satisfactorily. Mental distress can manifest itself in alcoholism, drug addiction, absenteeism, and suicidal tendencies that create hazards for both the affected individual and his co-workers. Also, the Vocational Rehabilitation Act of 1973 mandates that large federal contractors make an effort to hire qualified candidates who have physical disabilities or a history of mental illness.

The majority of company-sponsored counseling programs are headed by social workers rather than psychologists or psychiatrists. Successful programs have demonstrated that well-run counseling services can save the sponsoring company substantial amounts of money by reducing absenteeism, curbing hospital costs, and preventing the loss of valuable trained employees.

One of the most common counseling programs sponsored by industry is that to combat alcoholism and drug addiction. More than 2500 corporations have such programs. Alcoholism is a serious problem in industry, affecting the performance of many workers. It is estimated that 6 percent of the country's workforce have drinking problems. Company-sponsored programs have recovery rates of 60 to 80 percent, far higher than other programs that are not job-related. The reason for this phenomenon is coercion: a company can force an alcoholic to stick with a treatment program by threatening to fire him.

Many large corporations are creating broader programs to assist workers with all kind of problems from family conflicts to retirement planning. Although this consultation service may be viewed as another way of invading the privacy of the individual by big business, many employees voluntarily utilize the services when available and the results appear to be beneficial to all.

Stress in the workplace can also cause physical problems, such as ulcers, hypertension, and coronary artery disease. There are occupations that are subjected to much more stressful situations than others, and in this case cardiovascular monitoring is essential to assess the effects of the workplace on the employees, in spite of the fact that they are not exposed to hazardous agents.

Service companies that provide counseling for industrial clients charge between $1.00 to $1.50 per employee. It is estimated that each case that eventually ends up at the counseling service costs the sponsoring company anywhere between $80.00 and $130.00.

3
Chemical Substances Classified as Major Hazards

The variety and number of chemical agents found in the workplace boggles the mind. Attempts have been made to single out those substances that are particularly harmful to those handling them. This approach has produced standards and regulations for the handling of many chemical agents but has done little to devise medical surveillance techniques that are effective and preventive in nature. Currently, the trend is to eliminate separate classifications and regulations and to lump all agents into three basic categories, depending on their toxicity and health effects, and then to devise standard medical surveillance procedures for each category.

Whatever the future of the classification and regulation program, there are currently substances that are known to be potent health hazards and their handling poses special challenges for the manufacturer as he responds to the health needs of the work force. The deleterious effects of many of these substances have been verified by unnecessary human suffering, and the protection of the current work force has been the subject of extensive debate.

CARCINOGENS AND MUTAGENS

The identification of carcinogenic and mutagenic compounds in the work environment is a difficult and inexact task. Such identification is carried out by two basic methods:

animal experimentation, and
epidemiological studies of exposed human beings.

The validity of the extrapolation of results from animal experimentation to human beings has been questioned repeatedly. The basis of numerous objections to such a method of establishing the carcinogenicity of given compounds rests on the following observations:

> certain cancers are specific to certain species and do not affect others,
> animal exposure in the laboratory does not parallel human exposure in the working environment.

The physiological reactivity in animals and men of certain substances is well understood and in such cases, carcinogenicity in animals is easily related to carcinogenicity in human beings. Also, substances which attack a specific biological system, such as the lungs or gastrointestinal tract, appear to have similar results in "mice and men."

Epidemiological studies are crucial to the future of occupational medicine. Their role in understanding carcinogenicity in the industrial environment has been thwarted by the lack—sometimes purposeful—of proper record keeping; exacerbated the fact that in many cases industrial workers suffering from malignant disease have had varied exposures to a variety of substances.

OSHA has assumed that risk is directly correlated with level of exposure. Since it is widely accepted that carcinogenicity is closely dependent on exposure level and duration, research to pinpoint the degree of each of these necessary to induce cancer must be undertaken.

It has been estimated that there are approximately 2415 agents that are potentially carcinogenic. NIOSH investigators have some scientific evidence that these substances have potential carcinogenic activity in man, based on observations in human populations or experiments conducted on laboratory animals.

OSHA, in order to control and regulate employee exposure to carcinogens without having to prove the carcinogenicity of every potentially hazardous substance in the workplace, has devised a classification method that allows generalized grouping of toxic substances and generalized regulations and standards for each major group. The classification is as follows:

> *Category I Toxic Substance*: Potential occupational carcinogen in humans, or in two mammalian test species, or in a single mammalian species in two separate occasions, or in a single mammalian species if those results are supported by short-term tests, or if the Secretary is convinced that the substance belongs in this category.
>
> *Category II Toxic Substance*: Potential occupational carcinogen in studies in test humans or animals, the results of which tests are, however, found by the Secretary to be only suggestive. If verification is obtained, then this substance must be reclassified in Category I.
>
> *Category III Toxic Substance*: All toxic substances not classified in Category I or II and found in the American workplace.
>
> *Category IV Toxic Substance*: Any substance that would meet the definition of a toxic substance but is not currently found in the American workplace.

These classifications, first presented in 1977, were expected to be adopted in early 1980, after extensive hearings and debate, but have been withdrawn. The groupings will facilitate the establishment of medical surveillance standards, since many substances will be considered as a group rather than individually, allowing for a multiphasic screening approach.

A discussion of the mechanisms of establishing the carcinogenicity of industrial substances and standards development regarding exposure limits and worker protection is beyond the scope of this study. The emphasis is on the requirements for medical surveillance and the type of surveillance to be undertaken, that is, the nature of the medical examination and its frequency.

For the purposes of this report, we have attempted to identify major groups of industrial compounds that have proved or are suspected to be carcinogenic or mutagenic to illustrate the scope of the problem in the industrial sector and to estimate the degree of medical monitoring which will be required in the future to protect industrial workers. Medical surveillance is most important in this area because of the long latency period inherent in occupational carcinogenesis.

OSHA has developed a list of Class I toxic substances that includes both proved and suspected carcinogens. NIOSH is also continuously updating a list of hazardous substances, including carcinogens. The NIOSH list often specifies the organ site most vulnerable to the substances' cancer-causing effects and the type of medical monitoring necessary to obtain early signs of disease. These carcinogenic substances are listed in Table 2.

In this chapter, several agents that have proved to be carcinogenic in man, based on epidemiological studies, are discussed in some detail. OSHA medical surveillance requirements regarding exposure to such substances are also presented. There are many suspected carcinogens, as shown in Table 2, but detailed medical surveillance requirements have been established for only a few of these substances.

Asbestos

Asbestos refers to a group of fibrous silicate minerals with heat-resistant properties, and is in widespread use in the United States. The health effects of these materials have only just begun to manifest themselves, nearly 20 years after extensive exposure in asbestos mines, mills, and shipyards.

The problems created by asbestos stem from the fact that it is almost indestructable. It is not subject to decay or corrosion from acids, alkalies, or any chemicals. The fibers are needlelike and can continually break down into smaller and smaller fibers. Thus, the microscopic fibers are readily inhaled and from the lung they are carried to other parts of the body through the bloodstream. Because of their inert nature, there is a long latent period before disease develops, sometimes lasting as long as 50 years.

Table 2: Cancer Causing Substances*

	Kidney	Larynx Oral and Nasal	Leukemia	Liver	Skin	Urinary and Bladder	Cancer, Other
Acrylonitrile				?†			X† Gastrointestinal (GI) Tract
Aldrin/Dieldrin							
4-Aminobiphenyl						X	
Arsenic					X		X Lymphatic Pleural Cavity and GI Tract
Asbestos		X					
Auramine						?	
Benzene			X				? Lymphatic
Benzidine						X	? Pancreas
Beryllium							? Bone
Cadmium							X Prostate
Carbon black							X
Carbon tetrachloride				X			
Chloroform	X			X			
Chloroprene					?		?
Chromium		X					
Chrysene							X
Coal tar products					X		
Coke oven emissions	X						
DBCP							?
DDT				?			X

Major Chemical Hazards

Dioxane	?	
Ethylene dibromide	X	
Ethylene dichloride	X	
Ethylene oxide	X	
Ethylene thiourea	?	
Glycidyl ethers		
Heptachlor	X	
Hydrazines	X	
Isopropyl alcohol		?
Isopropyl oil		
Kepone		X
Lead	?	
Magenta		
4,4′-Methylene-bis	X	
Nickel carbonyl	X	
Nickel and compounds		X
4-Nitrodiphenyl		
O-Tolidine		
Pesticides, general	X‡	?
Polychlorinated biphenyls	X	X
Styrene butadiene	X	
Vinyl bromide	X	
Vinyl chloride	X	
Vinyl halides	X	

*A list of substances causing lung cancer is given in Table 5.
†An "X" signifies confirmed and a "?," suspected carcinogens.
‡Toxaphane.

Approximately one million tons of asbestos are used annually in the United States, mainly by the construction industry (insulation and acoustical products) and by manufactures in such areas as textiles, automobile (break linings and clutch facing), paper, paints, plastics, roof coatings, and floor tiles. Altogether, approximately 50,000 workers are involved in the manufacture of some 3000 asbestos-related products. An additional 40,000 field insulation workers are exposed to asbestos-containing products. However, nearly 3 to 5 million workers are exposed to asbestos on a secondary basis.

The health effects of asbestos exposure include: asbestosis, lung cancer, mesothelioma (pleural or peritoneal), and, to a lesser degree, other forms of cancer, such as that of the stomach, colon, and rectum. Additionally, because of the lightness of the fiber that is easily carried on clothing, families of workers are also affected with similar grave outcomes.

A recent epidemic of asbestos-related cancer in workers, 20 years after first exposure, resulted in recriminations, controversy, and litigation, but has not helped the quest for prevention of asbestos-related problems. Forecasters have estimated that the toll from asbestos-related cancers will exceed 1.6 million altogether, coming to about 58,000 to 75,000 deaths per year for the foreseeable future. This assumes that asbestos-related disease will continue to cause death at the same rate as before in spite of many atmospheric controls instituted by industry in the last 20 years.

In an effort to identify latent disease the government has begun a campaign to warn 11 million past and present asbestos workers, including 4.5 million World War II shipyard workers, of a possible lung cancer risk.

The asbestos exposure problem transcends conventional occupational risk, since it is thought to be a serious risk to the community at large. Asbestos mixed with other materials was sprayed onto interior building walls, from the mid 1940s until 1973, when the Environmental Protection Agency (EPA) banned this practice. As these surfaces began to deteriorate, asbestos fibers became airborne presenting a serious health hazard. Many older homes, schools, and other public buildings contain asbestos surfaces. Therefore the asbestos situation represents a problem beyond the scope of occupational medicine but is currently the responsibility of public health departments across the country.

OSHA medical surveillance standards require that all workers handling asbestos are given a preplacement examination that includes a medical history to elicit symptomatology of respiratory disease and pulmonary function tests. For workers exposed to asbestos for more than ten years or who are 45 years or older, a sputum cytology test is required. An annual examination must also be performed on all employees who come in contact with asbestos fibers incorporating all the tests included in the preplacement regimen. A similar examination must also be performed at termination of employment.

Recently the Consumer Product Safety Commission and the EPA issued a joint statement in which they said that human exposure to asbestos sources may present an unreasonable health risk to the general population. However, there is continuing controversy regarding the degree of exposure that is consistent with good health, and although progress is being made in the diagnosis and cure of occupational diseases, the asbestos case illustrates that the prevention of disease remains a political problem that has not yet been met.

Vinyl Chloride

Vinyl and polyvinyl chloride (PVC) are substances widely used in the manufacture of plastic products. Recently, in spite of the expectations of a recession, industry has been gearing up to expand production of PVC, which is second to polyethylene in volume among plastic resins. Total United States capacity is 7 billion pounds.

Vinyl chloride is a potent carcinogen affecting primarily the liver. OSHA standards recommend that all workers exposed to vinyl chloride undergo preassignment and annual and biannual examinations to assess any conditions of increased risk. The standard specifies that special attention be given to detecting enlargement of liver, spleen, or kidneys, or any dysfunction in these organs, and any abnormalities in skin, connective tissue, and the pulmonary system. The medical history should include the following:

alcohol intake,
past history of hepatitis and blood transfusions,
work history and past exposure to potential hepatotoxic agents, including drugs and chemicals, and
past history of hospitalizations.

Clinical laboratory tests to be performed include:

total bilirubin,
alkaline phosphatase,
serum glutamic oxalacetic transaminase (SGOT),
serum glutamic pyruvic transaminase (SGPT), and
gamma glutamyl transpeptidase (GGTP).

Additional tests that might be useful include: urine examinations for albumin, red blood cells, and exfoliated abnormal cells and such other serum tests as lactic acid dehydrogenase isoenzyme, protein determination, and protein electrophoresis. If abnormalities are detected in the serum evaluation, then a hepatitis B antigen test and liver scanning are recommended.

Although the primary concern over vinyl chloride exposure is its carcinogenic effects, this substance also causes nonmalignant alterations of the liver long before any malignancy becomes apparent. In addition to liver abnormalities, exposure to vinyl chloride has a toxic effect on the respiratory system and possible genetic effects. Also workers exposed to vinyl chloride appear to have an increased risk of developing hematopoietic and central nervous system tumors. Recently, it has been suggested that vinyl chloride is also a mutagen and a teratogen.

Petroleum and Petroleum Products (Benzene)

Increased cancer risk, especially cancers of the nasal cavity and sinuses, lung, and skin (melanoma), has been identified in the petroleum industry. A survey of cancer mortality conducted from 1950 to 1969 in countries with high concentrations of petroleum plants showed significantly higher cancer rates among male residents compared with control groups. It has been theorized that the increased risk is caused by exposure to polycyclic aromatic hydrocarbons (PAH) found in crude oil, in high boiling residues of catalytically cracked oils, in other pyrolysis products, in soots, and in the atmosphere around refining operations. Other occupations at risk from exposure to PAH include wax pressmen, workers in the shale oil industry, and mule spinners and machinists exposed to cutting oils. An increase in squamous cell cancers of the skin has been observed in this group. A high rate of melanoma was also noted among workers handling polychlorinated biphenyls. Lung cancer rates are also high among other PAH-exposed populations, such as roofers, coke oven workers, and gas generator employees.

Benzene, a product of petroleum processing, is also a suspected carcinogen, causing leukemia. Recently, OSHA proposed new exposure limits for benzene but the standard has been successfully contested in court by a suit filed by the American Petroleum Institute and 16 oil companies.

Benzene is widely used in the chemical industry for the manufacture of detergents, plastics, solvents, and paint removers. Approximately 11 billion pounds of benzene are produced annually and there are some 600,000 workers at 150,000 sites that are exposed to this substance.

Benzene commonly enters the body through the respiratory system, is rapidly diffused through the lungs, and is quickly absorbed into the blood and eventually accumulates in various body organs. It is subsequently metabolized by liver enzymes into water soluble derivatives and removed by the kidneys. It is theorized that it is the intermediates of the biotransformation of benzene, namely benzene epoxide, hydroquinone, and catechol, that exhibit the hematotoxic effects of benzene.

Exposure to high concentrations of benzene results in death. Lesser exposures produce nervous disturbances that often persist for weeks. Inhalation of still lower concentrations yields symptoms of mild poisoning that become rapidly reversible upon cessation of exposure. Also, direct contact with the liquid may cause erythema and blistering, with scaly dermatitis developing after repeated exposures.

The chronic effects of benzene exposure are not yet well understood. In general, benzene attacks the blood-forming systems, especially bone marrow. It causes alterations in the level of the formed elements (red cells, white cells, and platelets) of circulating blood that vary in severity from mild transient episodes to fatal disorders. Recently, research has also demonstrated that low level exposure to benzene causes chromosome damage, which, although in itself does not signify injury to workers, is usually an indication of an increased risk of cancer. One of the cancers most frequently detected in workers exposed to benzene is leukemia. Nonmalignant disorders include chronic anemia, low resistance to infections, impaired clotting of the blood, pancytopenia, and aplastic anemia. It has been reported that these types of blood disorders are generally reversible but can persist for long periods of time after cessation of exposure.

To date, the mechanism of chromosome damage or carcinogenicity caused by exposure to benzene has not been established. Also, no clear relationship has been discerned between exposure levels and cancer risk.

Benzene-induced leukemia is of the acute myelogenous type and has a poor prognosis with life expectancy of less than 6 months. Chronic leukemia has only occasionally been attributed to benzene exposure. A link between benzene exposure and chronic lymphocytic leukemia, a disease that occurs in late life, although suspected, has not been established.

The OSHA standard requires medical surveillance of only those employees who are exposed to benzene at or above the action level at employment and twice a year thereafter.

Exposure to PAHs has also been implicated in the increased incidence of gastrointestinal and bladder cancer among petroleum workers. However, epidemiological data have failed to show a cause-and-effect relationship.

Coke Oven Emissions

Coke oven emissions refer to the benzene-soluble fraction of total particulate matter present during the destructive distillation or carbonization of coal for the production of coke. These emissions are powerful carcinogens causing lung and kidney cancer and, if repeated exposure takes place, also skin cancer.

Coke is used as a fuel and reducing agent in blast furnace operations and in foundries as a cupola fuel. Approximately 61 million tons of coke are produced in the United States annually and 92 percent of this is used in blast furnaces, 5 percent in foundries, and 3 percent in other industrial operations. The steel industry produces more than 90 percent of the total coke volume with the remainder provided by foundries and beehive ovens.

The coking process involves many complex reactions resulting in emissions that contain a large number of recognized carcinogens as well as agents known to enhance the effect of carcinogens. Constituents of coke oven emissions include benzo(a)pyrene, benzo(b)fluoranthene, benzo(j)fluoranthene, benzo(b)anthracene, and chrysene, all carcinogens.

OSHA-mandated medical surveillance to be performed annually includes: a chest x-ray, pulmonary function tests, weight comparisons, skin examination, urinalysis (sugar, albumin, and hematuria), and urine and sputum cytology. The latter two tests are only recommended for workers older than the age of 45 years or those employed in the hazardous process for more than 5 years.

Arsenic

Arsenic is commonly present in various amounts (up to 6 percent) in sulfide ores mined for their copper, lead, zinc, gold, and silver content. Arsenic is also found in iron ore and coal. About 97 percent of arsenic enters the manufacturing process in the form of arsenic trioxide. Arsenic and its compounds are chiefly used in insecticides and herbicides. Other uses are found in glass production as a clarifying agent, in wood preservatives, and in drug production, electronics, textile printing, and tanning.

Compounds of arsenic include: lead arsenate, calcium arsenate, copper acetoarsenite, and magnesium arsenate.

Arsenic has been deemed a human carcinogenic based on epidemiological studies of exposed workers. Organ sites at risk are the respiratory and lymphatic systems. A study submitted to OSHA by the Dow Chemical Company showed that the cancer death rate among workers exposed to arsenic was high compared to that of a control group. Lung cancer deaths (16.2 percent) of the exposed population showed a threefold increase over the nonexposed group (5.7 percent). Lymphatic cancer occurred 2.5 times the expected rate (3.5 versus 1.4 percent). A study conducted by Allied Chemical also produced similar results. Although none of the findings has been verified, further studies conducted in other plants tend to substantiate them.

The medical surveillance recommendations set forth by OSHA cover all employees exposed to arsenic above the action level for at least 30 days per year. The surveillance standard includes a pre-employment examination by a physician, including medical and work history, to elicit any respiratory symptoms; x-rays, nasal and skin examination, sputum cytology, and other tests deemed desirable by the attending physician, and an annual examination for those above the age of 45 years and those exposed to arsenic for more than ten years.

Solvents and Chemical Intermediates

Hundreds of chemical intermediates are suspected carcinogens and it seems that new ones join the list with unrelenting regularity.

Acrylonitrile, a widely used chemical intermediate, is suspected to cause cancer in human beings. The United States produces approximately 1.5 billion pounds of this substance annually. Its major application is in the production of synthetic fibers. This substance has been found to be mutagenic, carcinogenic, and teratogenic in animals. Also, an epidemiological study carried out among exposed workers indicated an increased risk of lung cancer, with latent periods exceeding 20 years.

Acrylonitrile is also highly toxic, causing CNS, gastrointestinal, respiratory, and peripheral blood system disorders. It also causes dermatitis. Acute intoxication is fatal in many instances.

Medical surveillance requirements for those exposed to acrylonitrile on or above the action level include: a preplacement examination incorporating a medical and occupational history, with special attention to the skin, to respiratory and gastrointestinal systems, and to nonspecific symptoms, such as headache, nausea, vomiting, dizziness, and weakness; a complete physical examination, with special emphasis on the peripheral and central nervous systems, the gastrointestinal and respiratory systems, the skin, and the thyroid; a chest x-ray, and a fecal occult blood test for workers older than 40 years of age. The standard also requires periodic examinations and an examination at termination of employment.

Rules are also being written for other chemical intermediates suspected of carcinogenicity, such as epichlorohydrin, ethylene dichloride, and vinyl bromide.

Another substance suspected to be carcinogenic is ethylene oxide. Ethylene oxide is used in the production of ethylene glycol, in the manufacture of surface-active agents, as a fungicide and as a sterilant. United States production of ethylene oxide was nearly 4.5 billion pounds in 1972.

Ethylene oxide has been shown to be a mutagen in various organisms and is suspected to be carcinogenic in man. However, no adequate epidemiological studies exist to verify the carcinogenicity of this compound. One study performed in Sweden[22] showed an excess of leukemia incidence among workers exposed to ethylene oxide that methyl formate. The study, however, is not conclusive.

Other chemical intermediates, such as hydrazines, are also suspected of causing cancer. The NIOSH criteria document on these substances recommends that medical surveillance of employees exposed to these substances includes blood and urine tests, a chest x-ray, and for some workers bowel examinations. It is estimated that about 100,000 workers are exposed to hydrazines.

The National Cancer Institute (NCI) has also reported that EDC is a carcinogen, but any attempts to control the substance and produce health and safety standards regarding its use are far in the future. This agent is used in manufacturing vinyl chloride monomer from which PVC is made. About two million workers are exposed to EDC with about 33,675 getting full-time occupational exposure.

EDC is also used in textile dry cleaning, paint removers, and in making adhesives, such as rubber cement. Chemicals made from EDC include: Freon compounds, carbon tetrachloride, methyl chloroform, and perchloroethylene (dry cleaning solvent, most widely used). EDC enters the body by ingestion, inhalation, or skin absorption.

Pesticides and Herbicides

In addition to their toxic characteristics, many herbicides and pesticides are also suspected carcinogens. One of the pesticides newly confirmed as a carcinogen is toxaphene, one of the most widely used pesticides in the country, particularly on cotton crops, livestock, and produce. In 1976 the United States produced an estimated 100 million pounds of toxaphene. This pesticide has caused liver cancer and is also implicated in the development of thyroid cancer in laboratory animals.

TERATOGENS

Teratogenicity refers to functional or structural deviations evident at birth that can vary from minor abnormalities to catastrophic malformations. Agents act as teratogens when administered to either sex before mating, to the pregnant female, or directly to the fetus.

Mutagenesis, carcinogenesis, and teratogenesis are related phenomena and usually agents that cause one of these effects are also suspected of causing all of them.

Many environmental agents are known to affect negatively the course of pregnancy or cause fetal abnormalities. Agents such as alcohol, cigarette smoke, certain drugs, and radiation have been shown to affect the fetus. Occupational hazards in this area include many substances that are also considered toxic or carcinogenic.

The specter of the potential teratogenic effects of workplace substances haunts the employer and the government. Although it has been known for years that exposure to certain substances can cause sterility in men, it is still unclear how these substances affect the reproductive function of women. As more and more women enter the workplace, the importance of identifying teratogens becomes critical.

It is estimated that there are about 260,000 women employed in chemical plants. In the past, chemical companies refused employment to women of childbearing age to avoid the risk of huge liability claims. However, new laws prohibiting discrimination are forcing the companies to hire women and face up to the issue. Recently, women employees accused American Cyanamid of subjecting its workers to pressure and job placement discrimination when the company initiated a corporate program to insure the safety of women of childbearing age in its pigment plant where lead is used. The women faced imminent loss of well-paying jobs and transfer to less attractive janitorial positions unless they agreed to undergo a sterilization procedure. The company said that at no time did it suggest that the women submit to a sterilization procedure; on the contrary, it discouraged them from doing so.

However, the problem of health hazards arising from the manufacture of substances that are teratogenic or toxic transcends pregnant women and concerns both women of childbearing age and men. Many substances are mutagenic, with the potential of causing severe functional problems in offspring. Also, exposure to many chemical substances affects sperm production or results in sterility.

The problem with hazards in reproduction is that there are neither early warnings nor medical tests to monitor any health effects. On the other hand, there are huge liability risks, in the event of a damaged fetus, dreaded by both employer and insurer. The need is for more research to identify all major mutagens and teratogens in the workplace and guard against hazardous exposure levels.

A research program within the National Institute of Environmental Health Sciences (NIEHS) is concentrating on understanding the mechanisms of teratogenicity in humans and in identifying environmental teratogens. A project under contract to Dow Chemical and the Research Triangle Institute is attempting to determine the teratogenic potential of environmental agents in animals. NIEHS scientists are collaborating with the Endocrine Laboratories of Madison, Wisconsin, to screen selected environmental chemicals for transplacental toxicity. Chemicals under investigation include: zeranol, several polychlorinated biphenyls (PCB) and polybrominated biphenyls (PBB) isomers, DDE, and a series of mycotoxins. Effects on the male reproductive function are being evaluated in a contractual research effort with Hazelton Laboratories, which is assessing the reproductive toxicity of such metals as boron, cadmium, aluminum, and lead.

Substances with suspected teratogenic effects are listed in Table 6.

TOXIC SUBSTANCES

Toxic substances are defined as materials that are harmful to human beings. Their effects vary from mild transient discomfort to severe health problems that can even cause death. These substances, however, are not believed to be carcinogenic and the danger is usually related to accidental exposure. Many are critically hazardous in minute volumes, others tend to concentrate in vital organs and cause damage over longer time periods. Employee protection is usually provided by protective clothing and devices, strict adherence to hygiene, and to a lesser degree by medical monitoring.

Toxic substances usually enter the body via the respiratory route, although absorption through the skin is also possible.

The heaviest concentration of toxic substances is encountered in the chemical industry, where workers are exposed to thousands of substances, some of known but many of unknown toxicity. The variety and number of industrial toxic materials make it virtually impossible to discuss each separately. Therefore only some of the better known and widely used substances that cause chronic toxicity are discussed in some detail.

Pesticides and Herbicides

Pesticides and herbicides are a group of substances that are introduced into the environment to kill or injure some form of animal or plant life. These substances are extremely diverse in their chemical structure and in their toxic effects.

Pesticides and herbicides pose serious health problems not only to those associated with their production, but also to those who handle them (farmers, sprayers) and to the public at large.

There are 1200 pesticides registered with EPA and most of them are not regulated by OSHA, which has developed standards for only 180. In 1975, 1.61 billion pounds of pesticide active ingredients were produced in the United States and incorporated in more than 30,000 different products. Many of these substances are suspected carcinogens and most are potent human toxins when prolonged exposure occurs.

Approximately 8700 workers are employed in manufacturing and formulating facilities that primarily produce pesticides. Also, there are 350,000 employees who are potentially exposed because they work at plants that produce pesticides as secondary products.

NIOSH has issued criteria for a recommended standard on occupational exposure to pesticides. OSHA intends to issue a standard based on broad categories rather than a substance-by-substance approach. Substances are to be classified in three groups according to their toxicity (such a classification has already been established by the EPA) and each group is to be regulated separately.

The intended standard will also include medical surveillance requirements, such as preplacement and periodic examinations. The screening emphasis is to be concentrated in examining the eyes, liver, kidneys, lungs, and the peripheral nervous system. Special screening procedures have not as yet been suggested.

The dangers of pesticide exposure were brought into focus by the Kepone incident, a case in which employees were exposed to dangerous levels of the pesticide Kepone and later developed serious neurological and other disorders, such as sterility. In this case the cause of the problem was incredible negligence on the part of the employer.

Kepone can be absorbed through the skin, and the company issued rubber gloves but did not inform the workers of the danger. Therefore the workers did not wear the gloves and continued to eat their lunches at the workbenches, and to carry the dust home on their clothes. In a relatively short time, the workers began to complain of memory loss, trembling hands, slurred speech, and chest and abdominal pain. Some also became sterile. Tests disclosed liver, spleen, and brain damage. Although most of the symptoms have been reversed, scientists are monitoring the workers to assess the long-term effects of the exposure for carcinogenicity or other complications.

Several pesticides have been deemed dangerous by environmental protection agencies. Recently, an administrative law judge decided that the EPA should ban dibromochloropropane (DBCP), which causes sterility and cancer in exposed workers. Subsequently the EPA suspended nearly all uses of DBCP except in Hawaiian pineapple groves.

Another potentially harmful pesticide is endrin, which is suspected of causing birth defects. Some 175,000 kg. of endrin are used on cotton, wheat, and apple crops annually in the United States.

Herbicides are also expected to come under scrutiny in the future. Many such substances are suspected of causing toxicity in human beings. One example of a potent toxin found as a contaminant in commercial samples of a commonly used herbicide, 2,4,5-trichlorophenoxyacetic acid, is contaminated with a dioxin that is often referred to as TCDD (2,3,7,8-tetrachlorodibenzo-p-dioxin). Dioxin was also a component of "agent orange," a defoliant used in Vietnam. Vietnam War veterans have complained of serious health problems as a result of ingesting dioxin; some may have died from it. The case against dioxin is not settled yet because a recent study by Monsanto involving 121 workers believed to have been exposed to TCDD in an industrial accident 30 years ago did not disclose any increase in mortality from cancer or cardiovascular disease. This study is an ongoing evaluation of workers who were employed in the 2,4,5-T operations at Monsanto.

In the spring of 1981 the American Council on Science and Health (ACSH) issued a position paper based on a review of the scientific evidence regarding 2,4,5-T. It was their conclusion that there is insufficient evidence to indicate a relationship between the traditional use of 2,4,5-T and adverse health effects in human beings. ACSH recommended that the substance be used in rice fields, rangelands, forests, along railways and highways, and in landscaping.

Another herbicide, Oryzalin, is suspected of causing birth defects among the children of workers exposed to this agent.

Metals and their Compounds

Metals enter the body via the inhalation of dusts or fumes and in a few cases by absorption through the skin. Metals and their compounds abound in industry. Among those suspected to be detrimental to human health or under investigation, are: aluminum, antimony, arsenic, beryllium, cadmium, cobalt, copper, indium, iron, lead, lithium, magnesium, manganese, mercury, nickel, palladium, phosphorus, platinum, selenium, silver, thallium, tungsten, and zinc.

Many of these metallic substances are extremely toxic, with exposure occurring in metal mining, refining, fabrication, and cleaning applications. Two proved toxic metals, lead and beryllium, are discussed below in some detail.

Cadmium has been shown to cause nephrotoxicity and affect pancreatic function. This metal is extremely toxic in acute exposure, causing severe pulmonary edema. Long-term problems after exposure include emphysema and liver damage.

Particularly vulnerable to metal toxicity is the hematopoietic system. Exposure to selenium, vanadium, arsenic, and lead causes anemia, whereas other metals, such as antimony and manganese, are implicated in leukopenia.

Mercury vapors cause CNS changes, including depression, insomnia, memory loss, tumor, and peripheral neuropathy. Exposure to mercury compounds also causes such serious problems as nerve, brain, and kidney damage. Mercury toxicity is also implicated in the development of glomerulonephritis and erethism, a form of anxiety neurosis, is almost specific for chronic occupational exposure. It is theorized that mercury and other heavy metals can induce autoimmune diseases resulting in the formation of antigen/antibody complexes.

The therapeutic use of mercury, as a diuretic and cathartic, as a disinfectant, and as a treatment for venereal disease, has greatly decreased.

Lead. In the United States, industry consumes in excess of 1 million tons of lead yearly and potential exposure to lead occurs in at least 120 occupations, including manufacture of lead storage batteries and automobiles, ship building and repair, brass and bronze foundries, steel producing, lead pigment users and manufacturers, lead smelting, ceramic and glass working, soldering, babbiting, metal burning, painting, plumbing, working with scrap and sheet metal, and printing. A new occupational hazard has also been created by the requirements set forth in many states to delead old houses and public places.

Some of the potential hazards of lead poisoning have been known since the ancient Greeks. Recently OSHA published a new standard that limits worker exposure to 50 mg/m^3 in air, from the heretofore accepted 200 mg/m^3 level. The total cost of compliance with this standard has been estimated at $3.25 billion in the next decade and there is doubt if technology is available to aid industry in complying with this standard in all cases.

Acute effects of severe lead inhalation include: damage to the CNS, which is impossible to reverse, as well as damage to the kidneys and the reproductive system. Long-term exposure causes damage to the nervous system, especially to the neuromuscular and psychomotor functions. Low-level exposure may also increase the risk of contracting a number of chronic diseases, such as hypertension and nephritis.

Lead exposures cause greater harm in certain worker groups, such as female workers of childbearing age and those having anemia or renal insufficiency. Also, persons with the sickle cell trait may be subjected to a greater risk.

The medical surveillance program for exposed workers requires that:

> a preplacement physical examination is performed that includes: a complete medical and occupational history, a complete blood count and routine

urinalysis (specific gravity, sugar, protein determinations, and microscopic examinations), and a pregnancy test when appropriate,
annual examinations for all exposed workers are performed, and
blood lead level monitoring is carried out every two months for employees with blood lead levels greater than 40 μg/100 gm of whole blood

The biological monitoring program, aimed to insure that workers are not exposed to dangerous lead levels, relies on lead concentrations in the blood of workers at risk. Blood testing can be replaced by urine sampling and analysis. If abnormal results are obtained, biological monitoring must be carried out at close intervals until the blood lead level drops below the maximum allowable by the regulations.

Biological testing methods to identify hazardous lead exposure workplaces are described in chapter 8 of this study.

Beryllium. Beryllium is a light metal used extensively in industry as an alloy. It is used in the manufacture of ceramic parts, household appliances, electric circuitry, electrical measuring instruments, thermal coatings, switch-gear, and welding apparatus. It also is used in the aerospace and nuclear industries in the manufacture of inertial guidance systems, rocket motor parts and fuels, aircraft brake systems, gyroscopes, heat shields, and moderator reflectors.

Exposures to dusts and fumes containing beryllium may occur in both large-scale processing plants and in small plants that perform such operations as melting, casting, grinding, drilling, and machining.

Domestic production of beryl, the principal beryllium-containing ore of commercial importance, was approximately 500 tons in 1950. Domestic production has remained relatively constant as contrasted with domestic consumption, which, in 1969, reached 8500 tons and is expected to reach 20,000 tons by the year 2000. A survey conducted by the United States Public Health Service in 1970 estimated that 30,000 persons in the work force could have potential exposure to dust or fumes containing beryllium.

Beryllium is extremely toxic, with both acute and chronic manifestations of disease. Also, it is a suspected carcinogen, mostly affecting the respiratory tract. The carcinogenicity of beryllium remains a speculation but its toxicity was confirmed in the 1950s.

Acute effects include dermatitis, ulcers, and various ocular disturbances. Abscesses and ulcerations result from crystal implantation of beryllium materials in cutaneous areas previously injured by cuts or abrasions. Ocular effects include inflammation of the conjunctiva, and corneal burns. Beryllium-induced acute respiratory effects range from a mild inflammation of the nasal mucous membranes and pharynx to severe pneumonitis.

Chronic beryllium-caused disease often does not manifest itself until several years after the last exposure and it is characterized as a systemic disorder of prolonged duration and progressive in severity despite cessation of exposure. Its most familiar symptom is pneumonitis. Other systemic effects include heart enlargement leading to cardiac failure, enlargement of the liver and spleen, cyanosis, and kidney stones.

A Beryllium Case Registry instituted in 1952 at Massachusetts General Hospital in Boston recorded 893 cases by 1981 and about 10 to 12 new cases are added every year.

Medical surveillance requirements include a preemployment examination consisting of the following:

> a medical and occupational history,
> determination of any respiratory symptoms,
> chest x-rays,
> pulmonary function tests,
> baseline weight, and
> a skin examination.

An annual examination is also recommended for all exposed individuals.

Solvents and Chemical Intermediates

Solvent byproducts enter the body mainly via the respiratory tract but are also absorbed through the skin. There are many different types of solvents used in industry, presenting a wide range of hazards. Some of the common solvents, such as benzol (benzene), carbon tetrachloride, carbon disulfide, and methanol, are highly toxic and must be used under strictly controlled conditions.

There are thousands of chemical solvents and intermediates and many have toxic effects on human beings. Regulations have been written for many such intermediates and new rules are being formulated continuously. Standards in place exist for many substances, such as ketones (alkylbenzens, toluene, trichloroethylene). Ketones are toxic to the liver, the kidney, and the nervous system. The medical surveillance requirements only refer to preexisting conditions and complaints after exposure. NIOSH requires urinalysis of exposed workers.

Exposure to p-tert-butytoluene, an alkyl benzene, also requires such medical surveillance as preplacement and periodic tests. This substance affects the cardiovascular and hematopoietic systems. Recommended tests, in addition to a medical history and a physical examination, include an electrocardiogram (EKG) and a complete blood count (differential count, hemoglobin, hematocrit, and clotting time).

Trichloroethylene, a common solvent, is also considered highly toxic, affecting many diverse body systems. Exposure to this agent causes CNS depression, visual disturbances, mental confusion, cardiac fibrillation, and liver and kidney effects. Chronic exposure may produce double vision and even blindness. Other effects include loss of the olfactory and impairment of the tactile sense. Trichloroethylene is also suspected to be carcinogenic.

Medical surveillance requirements include preplacement and periodic examinations. The preplacement examination includes the following tests:

- a medical history, including information on cardiac and pulmonary problems, seizure disorders, liver disease, incidences of headache, nausea and dizziness, eye problems, irritation of mucous membranes, skin irritation, and
- a physical examination which must include a general physical examination, an EKG, urinalysis, pulmonary function tests, and a complete blood count.

Toluene, another solvent, is also considered toxic at prolonged exposure. Most of toluene is used in the manufacture of benzene and other chemicals. NIOSH estimates that 100,000 workers or more could have potential exposure to toluene, production of this substance recently being more than a million gallons.

Toluene causes skin and eye irritation. High exposure also affects the CNS and hematopoietic systems. Medical surveillance requirements include both preplacement and periodic examinations. The preplacement examination is similar to the one described for trichloroethylene, except that no EKG is recommended.

NIOSH has also prepared criteria documents for other chemical intermediates, such as benzyl chloride and glycidyl ethers.

Benzyl chloride causes eye, skin, and upper respiratory irritation. Approximately 90 million pounds of the compound are produced in the United States annually. NIOSH estimates that 3000 workers are exposed to this agent. NIOSH recommends chest x-rays and pulmonary function tests for exposed workers.

NIOSH estimates that 118,000 workers are exposed to glycidyl ethers and that an additional one million workers are exposed to epoxy resins in which the glycidyl ethers are used as diluents. Exposure to these agents causes dermatitis, sensitization, irritation, and allergic reactions.

GASES

Dangerous gases encountered in the occupational environment include: carbon monoxide, hydrogen sulfide, hydrogen fluoride, hydrogen cyanide, methyl bromide, chlorine, ozone, nitrogen dioxide, nitrous oxide, and sulfur dioxide.

Gases are present in the work environment either as a result of chemical processes or by accident, such as in leaks, incomplete combustion, and improper ventilation. The health effects can range from minor headaches and eye irritation to asphyxiation.

Carbon monoxide, a highly toxic gas, poisons by displacing oxygen in the blood and it can kill within minutes. Small quantities can cause headaches, dizziness, nausea, drowsiness, and inattention. Long-term exposure may also cause permanent damage to heart and brain tissue.

Sulfur dioxide is a colorless, irritant gas formed during the combustion of sulfur. The gas is widely used in a variety of industries and is a common workplace hazard. It exerts its toxic influences through both acute and chronic effects. Acute symptoms are eye and upper respiratory irritation. Chronic effects include: nasopharyngitis, reduction of pulmonary function, and perhaps promotion of cancer. OSHA recommends that medical surveillance of affected workers should include x-ray and pulmonary function tests as well as eye and skin examinations. These tests are to be performed annually on all individuals exposed to sulfur dioxide above the action level. Overall, it is estimated that 500,000 workers are exposed to sulfur dioxide.

Ozone, another potentially toxic gas, is extremely irritating to the upper and lower respiratory tract. Ozone and nitrogen dioxide are contributing, if not primary, causes of pulmonary emphysema and chronic nonspecific pulmonary disease. Ozone may also cause local irritation of the eyes and mucous membranes. At high exposure it can cause pulmonary edema. Systemically, it mimics the effects of ionizing radiation and may therefore cause chromosomal damage.

OSHA recommends that workers exposed to ozone undergo preplacement and periodic medical examinations. The preplacement examination consists of a medical history and a physical examination with emphasis on the respiratory system. Special tests include pulmonary (forced vital capacity [FVC] and forced expiratory volume in one second [FEV_1]), and a chest x-ray. The employer must also provide access to the physician in case a worker complains of any symptoms associated with ozone exposure.

The use of nitrous oxide for dental procedures puts dentists, dental assistants, and other office personnel at risk, although long-term effects have not been clearly established. There are no known short-term effects from inhalation by patients. It is estimated that some 47,000 dentists use the gas in their practices, and circulating gas in the air of the dental office can reach as high as 8000 parts per million.

NIOSH has recommended to OSHA that a maximum occupational level of 50 ppm be established, although dental authorities consider this level to be too low for practical purposes and maintain that it should at least be double that number.

Adverse health effects of occupational exposure to nitrous oxide include increased incidence of liver and kidney cancers and spontaneous abortion in women and a greater number of birth defects in offspring born to workers of both sexes.

DUSTS

Most dusts encountered in the work environment are biologically inert and simply a nuisance. There are, however, many types of dusts that are extremely hazardous. The hazard depends on the composition of the dust, the size of the dust particles, and the duration of exposure.

Dusts that are harmful are those that contain free silica (silicon dioxide not chemically bound) found in quartz, granite, flint, sandstone and sand. Other harmful dusts include cotton, coffee, cottonseed and coal. Asbestos, as discussed elsewhere, is similarly harmful.

Dusts mainly affect the respiratory system. Disorders caused by hazardous dusts include asthma, pulmonary fibrosis, byssinosis, and industrial bronchitis. These disabling chronic diseases take a long time to become symptomatic and are often irreversible when discovered. Monitoring workers exposed to hazardous dusts is therefore of the utmost importance. Some dust inhalation is immediately toxic, however, such as graphite dust.

Cotton Dust

Cotton production in the United States averages between 10 and 13 million bales. The cotton industry can be divided into 11 major processes: (1) harvesting; (2) ginning; (3) warehousing and compressing of cotton lint; (4) classing and marketing of cotton lint; (5) yarn manufacturing using cotton lint; (6) fabric manufacturing using cotton yarn; (7) reclaiming and marketing of textile manufacturing waste; (8) delintering of cottonseed; (9) marketing and converting of linters; (10) reclaiming and marketing of gin motes; and (11) batting, yarn, and felt manufacturing using waste cotton fibers and byproducts. Within each of these major processes there are various stages, distinct work procedures, and methods of operation. The states that are the largest producers of cotton are Texas, California, Mississippi, and Arkansas; the textile industry is concentrated in the south.

Cotton dust causes a serious lung disease called byssinosis, or brown lung disease. It is estimated that approximately 35,000 textile workers, employed and retired, are currently disabled because of this disease. Additionally there are thousands of nontextile workers exposed to dust that are disabled. Recently, OSHA proposed a standard limiting worker exposure to cotton dust. The industry challenged the standard in the federal appeals court but it was upheld by the court. The standard applies to textile operations such as preparation and yard departments and weaving and for such nontextile operations as cottonseed oil plants. About 600,000 workers are exposed to cotton dust. Each of these two industries is to comply to different exposure limit standards, including some variations in medical surveillance requirements.

Medical surveillance requirements of workers exposed to cotton dust in the textile industry, as set forth by OSHA, are as follows:

    initial examination, including a medical history using a standardized questionnaire, pulmonary function tests (FVC and FEV_1 and their departure from normal values) and a grading according to the risk of the employee to acquire byssinosis,

annual examinations, including an updated medical history and pulmonary function tests, and
biennial examination of those workers that exhibit: an FEV_1 of greater than 80 percent of predicted but an FEV_1 decrement of 5 percent or 200 ml on a first working day, an FEV_1 of less than 80 percent of the predicted value, or other symptoms deemed significant by the attending physician.

Medical surveillance requirements for those exposed to cotton dust in cotton gins are similar to those just discussed, except that OSHA requires a mid-season retest, similar to the one performed at the time of worker placement, to be performed after at least 14 days of employment and before termination of employment for the season.

Coal Dust

It has been known for years that coal dust causes severe pulmonary disorders. Affected individuals are primarily mine workers. Mining has been traditionally a very hazardous occupation but in recent years safety standards promulgated by the government and adopted by industry have eliminated many of the accident risks associated with this occupation. In 1981 a reversal of this trend began.

Health risks remain a problem. The most common problem encountered in coal mining is a respiratory disorder, pneumoconiosis, otherwise known as black lung disease. Estimates place the incidence of this disease among coal miners at 4 to 11 percent, depending on the geographical location of the mine. Therefore this is a common disorder that could become even more significant in the future as the United States turns to coal for its energy needs.

Health and safety regulations in mining are put forth by a separate government agency established by the Coal Miner Safety and Health Act. This agency requires that all coal miners are monitored periodically by x-ray and pulmonary function tests.

EYE AND SKIN IRRITANTS

Skin problems account for more than 46 percent of all reported occupational illnesses. Skin disorders range from simple irritation to serious dermatitis and are often an indication of improper prophylactic and hygiene practices. Numerous substances cause skin irritation, as listed in Table 3.

The most common skin effect is eczematous dermatitis which accounts for more than 75 percent of all occupationally induced dermatoses. About 20 percent of occupational dermatitis is caused by allergic sensitization.

Nearly every occupational group is exposed to agents that may produce skin effects. Skin problems can be prevented by installing environmental controls, supplying workers with personal protective devices, such as gloves or creams, and by avoiding contact with irritating substances.

Often the presence of skin problems may be the precursor of serious systemic disease caused by exposure to toxic agents.

Eye injuries and disorders are also common in industry with 130,000 such incidents reported in 1975. Substances that cause eye irritation and damage are also listed in Table 3.

Table 3: Substances Causing Eye and Skin Irritation

Substance	Condition
Acetic acid	Eye and skin irritant
Acids and alkalis	Dermatitis
Acrylamide	Skin and eye irritant
Acrylonitrile	Skin irritant
Alkanes	Skin irritant
Allyl alcohol	Eye and skin irritant
Ammonia	Eye damage if contact
Amyl alcohol	Eye and skin irritant
Aniline	Eye irritant
Antimony	Skin and eye irritant, dermatitis
Arsenic	Dermatitis
Asphalt fumes	Eye irritant
Benzene	Dermatitis, erythema, eye irritant
Benzoyl peroxide	Eye and skin irritant
Benzyl chloride	Eye and skin irritant
Beryllium	Dermatitis, skin abscesses and ulcerations, ocular inflammation of the conjuctiva, corneal burns.
Boron hydrides	Skin irritant
Brass	Dermatitis
Bromine and hydrogen bromide	Eye and skin irritant
Carbon black	Skin irritant
Chlorine	Eye irritant
Chlorinated naphthalene or diphenyl compounds	Dermatitis
Chromium	Skin ulcers
Cresol	Skin and eye irritant
DBCP	Erythema, dermatitis
Dinitro-ortho-cresol	Eye and skin irritant
Dioxane	Skin irritant
Ethylene dibromide	Eye and skin irritant
Ethylene oxide	Sensitization and irritation of the skin
Fibrous glass	Eye and skin effects

(Table 3: continued overleaf)

Table 3: continued

Substance	Condition
Glycidyl ethers	Skin irritant
Hydrazines	Eye and skin effects
Hydrogen fluoride	Skin and eye irritant
Hydrogen sulfide	Irritation of the eyes
Hydroquinone	Eye and skin irritant
Methyl alcohol	Blindness
Microwave radiation	Cataracts
Nickel and compounds	Skin irritant
Organotin compounds	Skin effects
Phenol	Skin and eye effects
Plant products	Allergic skin reactions
Polychlorinated biphenyls	Skin effects
Solvents	Dermatitis
Sulfur oxide	Eye irritant
Synthetic resins	Dermatitis
Thiols	Eye and skin irritant
Toluene diisocyanate	Skin irritant
Tungsten and cemented tungsten carbide	Skin effects
Vanadium	Eye and skin effects

4
Environmentally Induced Diseases and Disorders

Numerous diseases and disorders have their etiology in environmental exposure factors. Also, workplace hazards can act as triggering mechanisms in the manifestation of many health problems. Both chronic and acute health problems are encountered, often complicated by the fact that many diseases do not appear until years after exposure.

Probably the most dreaded health problem currently attributed to environmental factors is cancer. Manifestations of this disease often do not appear until after long latent periods, complicating attempts to use epidemiologic methodology to assess the carcinogenic effects of the myriads of chemical products in the market today.

Although cancer is uppermost on everyone's list, other disorders, such as pulmonary disease, liver disease, reproductive dysfunction, and skin and eye irritation, also challenge the health of the industrial worker. Many of the disorders are preventable and often reversible if detected in their early stages. For many, medical screening techniques have been developed that permit early detection. Others, however, can only be detected after considerable damage has occurred and when reversal is impossible.

Considered below are some of the more serious and more prevalent diseases that threaten the health of industrial workers.

CANCER

The problem with occupationally induced diseases such as cancer is that they do not manifest themselves immediately but rather develop over long periods of time and become symptomatic years after the first exposure occurred. Also, carcinogens exist in nearly all environments and total avoidance is impossible. However, these carcinogens often become significant if they exist in a certain concentration, over a particular period of time, and in conjunction with other environmental conditions. Therefore pinpointing the effect of carcinogens in the atmosphere or the work place is sometimes problematic.

Exposure to carcinogens is all too commonplace. Also, other factors, such as dietary and personal habits, smoking, and genetic predispositions, although potentially carcinogenic in themselves, become doubly hazardous when an individual is simultaneously exposed to industrial carcinogens.

NIOSH has published a study[50] that has estimated the relative risks of developing specific forms of cancer in subjects engaged in various occupations. The results of the study are based on a data base of patients admitted to a single medical research and treatment facility, Roswell Park Memorial Institute, Buffalo, New York. The project spanned the years 1956 to 1965 and involved 25,416 individuals with 22 different kinds of cancer. More than 8943 different occupations were represented in the patient sample. Overall, an increased incidence of certain types of cancer among given groups of industrial workers was discerned.

Environmentally induced cancer is also a public health hazard affecting the population near plants producing dangerous substances. Industrial states, such as New Jersey, report higher cancer death rates than other less industrialized states. Actually, New Jersey, with a 1977 cancer death rate of 203.1 per 100,000, nearly 15 percent higher than the national average, adopted new antipollution regulations to set curbs on carcinogens. Substances to be regulated include asbestos, benzene, carbon tetrachloride, chloroform, dioxane, ethylenimine, ethylene dibromide, ethylene, dichloride, 1, 1, 2, 2-tetrachloroethane, tetrachloroethylene, 1,1,1-trichloroethane, and trichloroethylene.

Leukemia

Leukemia is cancer of the white blood cells. It is characterized by abnormal immature cells in the circulating blood, a replacement of bone marrow by malignant cells, and infiltrates in the liver and spleen and other tissues. Leukemia is classified as acute or chronic and, depending on the type of cells affected, as myeloid, monocytic, or lymphoid.

The most prevalent leukemia types among adults and the ones commonly associated with exposure to workplace hazards are acute myeloid leukemia and acute myeloblastic leukemia. Most acute myelogenous leukemias have a poor prognosis with life expectancies ranging from 6 to 18 months.

Several industrial agents, as shown in Table 2, are suspected of causing leukemia. Other hazardous substances also attack the hematopoietic system and cause related abnormalities, such as various types of anemias.

Medical screening for leukemia is by hematological evaluation.

Lung Cancer

Lung cancer accounts for about 14 percent of all cancer deaths in the United States. Cigarette smoking is the predominant cause of lung cancer, but many industrial agents also cause or are suspected of causing lung cancer, as can be seen in Table 4. Actually, more carcinogens affect the lung than any other organ. Occupational hazards coupled with smoking further increase the risk of contracting lung cancer among industrial workers.

The incidence of lung cancer from occupational causes appears to be proportional to the dose and duration of exposure to the responsible carcinogen. Industrial susceptibility is further modified by genetic predisposition, immune factors, underlying respiratory disease, and personal habits, such as smoking.

Lung cancer risks among occupational workers were brought into focus with the recent discovery of the disease in workers who handled asbestos during their employment. OSHA recommended medical surveillance of asbestos workers consisting of the following steps:

Preplacement Examination. Chest x-ray, medical history to identify pre-existing respiratory disease, and pulmonary function tests (FVC and FEV_1).

Annual Examination. A comprehensive medical examination, including at least a chest x-ray, a medical history, and pulmonary function tests.

Table 4: Agents Suspected of Causing Lung Cancer

Confirmed	Suspected
Acrylonitrile	Beryllium
Arsenic, inorganic	Cadmium
Asbestos	Chloroprene
Bis (chlomethyl) ether	Iron oxide
Carbon black	Lead
Chloroethyl methyl ether	Nitrous oxide
Chromates	
Chromium (VI)	
Chrysene	
Coal tar products	
Coke oven emissions	
Mustard gas	
Nickel and its compounds	
Radon	
Silica	
Uranium	
Vinyl chloride	

Termination of Employment Examination. Similar tests as in periodic screening.

Maintenance of Medical Records. Records must be maintained for 20 years.

This screening regimen could be considered as a standard for workers exposed to carcinogens suspected of causing lung cancer. It is generally accepted that x-rays are potentially useful methods of detecting presymptomatic lung cancer. Another screening technique, sputum cytology, is also used in the early detection of cancer. Both these techniques must be applied with extreme care and evaluated by experts, if they are to be at all useful as screening methods. Other methods of lung cancer detection include bronchoscopy, biochemical markers, immunological testing, and hormonal factors. However, most of these techniques are only practical when the patient presents himself with symptoms that indicate serious disease.

Although screening for lung cancer appears possible with currently available techniques, there is no proof that such screening has any effect on mortality from the disease. The NCI sponsored a *Consensus Conference on Screening for Lung Cancer* in September 1978 to determine whether currently available screening tests give evidence of reducing mortality from lung cancer among high-risk individuals. The recommendations of the conference were as follows:

> Current prospective studies of asymptomatic individuals who have been screened for lung cancer by chest x-ray examination and sputum cytology do not at present show any evidence of a significant reduction in mortality from the disease. These studies must be continued for several more years before the accumulated information will be sufficient to allow a relationship between screening and mortality to be determined. Results of these studies should be kept under continuing review.
>
> Until the value of screening for lung cancer by these methods has been demonstrated, mass screening programs should be limited to well-designed, controlled studies, with provision for analysis of results, and for further diagnostic work-up and treatment, when indicated.
>
> Although some screening programs for lung cancer have been initiated among workers in certain industries, caution is strongly recommended in starting any new ones. Screened workers cannot be assured of an overall benefit on the basis of existing data.
>
> None of these recommendations on the application of chest radiography and sputum cytology in screening are intended to apply to their diagnostic use in individuals who present to physicians signs or symptoms that suggest lung cancer.
>
> Continued research on better methods of screening for lung cancer, including improvements in the methods now under trial, should be strongly supported. At present, no other techniques appear to be ready for clinical application.

Whether for screening or diagnosis, the control of quality in performing and interpreting chest radiography and sputum cytology is essential.

Since screening by current methods is unlikely to solve the problem of lung cancer control, strenuous efforts should be devoted to primary prevention. The greatest reduction in mortality can be achieved by cessation of cigarette smoking, with additional important benefits from reduction of exposure to other respiratory carcinogens (environmental and occupational). Elimination of combined exposure to cigarette smoke and other airborne carcinogens is particularly important because their effects on lung cancer incidence are often synergistic.

Other Cancers

Several rare types of cancer also occur almost exclusively due to occupational exposure. One such cancer is mesothelioma, a diffuse malignancy of the lining of the lungs and the peritoneum. This type of malignancy has a dismal prognosis, with death occurring usually within a year of diagnosis. Mesothelioma is an extremely rare cancer with an incidence of two cases per million per year, and is related to asbestos exposure.

Cancer of the pancreas is now one of the leading causes of death from malignant neoplasms but no environmental factors contributing to its incidence have been identified. Cigarette smoking, genetic and environmental factors are suspected but have not been confirmed. Occupational groups considered at risk to develop this cancer include chemists, workers exposed to aromatic amines, metal workers, and aluminum millers. NIOSH only lists cresol as a hazard particularly affecting the pancreas. Also beryllium is suspected to be a pancreatic carcinogen.

Esophageal, oral, and nasal cancers are also quite common in the United States. Smoking is the single most important environmental determinant in esophageal and oral cancers. Table 2 lists some of the industrial hazards associated with such cancers. Esophageal cancer incidence is elevated in workers exposed to asbestos. Nasal cancer (adenocarcinomas) is found at high rates among furniture workers.

Oral cancers have been found in excessive rates among male and female textile and apparel industry workers. However, smoking and orally taken snuff are probably responsible for the majority of environmentally induced oral cancers.

Brain tumors have also been associated with occupational exposure to workplace carcinogens. Increased incidence of brain cancer has been associated with workers in the petroleum industry.

Cancer of the prostate, a common malignancy in men, has also been associated with occupational exposures. One agent suspected of causing cancer of the prostate is cadmium. Higher incidences of cancer of the prostate have been encountered in the rubber industry. Also, higher rates of prostate cancer were encountered in counties with metal-using and textile industries. However, no study has developed a direct link between prostate cancer and industrial exposures.

Cancer of the gastrointestinal tract is also suspected of being caused by exposure to industrial agents. However, other factors, such as ethnicity and nutritional habits, seem to play a far more important role than industrial carcinogens.

Cancer of the liver has been associated with exposures to vinyl chloride.

Many substances, such as aromatic amines, benzidine, alpha-naphthylamine, beta-naphthylamine, and nitro-biphenyl, are also suspected of causing bladder cancer. Workers in the chemical, rubber, and printing industries are believed to be at risk.

RESPIRATORY DISEASE

Respiratory disease is a common complication of exposure to occupational irritants and toxins. Lung cancer, a grave complication relating to occupational exposures, has been discussed above. In this section other respiratory diseases, reversible and irreversible, are discussed as they relate to occupational exposure. Numerous agents assault the respiratory system, as is shown in Table 5.

One of the most important contributors to respiratory disease is cigarette smoking. In high-risk occupations workers who smoke stand a higher probability of contracting respiratory disease than those who do not. Pulmonary assessment is critical in such cases, for early signs of deterioration can be identified and major irreversible disease prevented.

Interestingly, genetic susceptibility is also a significant factor. Familial respiratory disease can be used as an indication of added risk. Genetic predesposition is also evident in those with $alpha_1$-antitrypsin deficiency.

Respiratory disease caused by occupational exposures includes: asthma, hypersensitivity pneumonitislike syndrome, hemorrhagic pneumonia, interstitial pneumonitis, pulmonary granulomas, pulmonary fibrosis, pneumoconiosis, sarcoidosis, byssinosis, industrial bronchitis, and silicosis. Diseases are known by such descriptive names as "black lung," "brown lung," "farmers lung," and "pigeon breeders disease."

The government is funding several major efforts to study the causes and mechanisms of occupationally induced respiratory disease. Funding agencies include the NIEHS, through its Inhalation Toxicology Section and the National Heart, Lung and Blood Institute (NHLBI) through its Fibrotic and Immunologic Pulmonary Diseases Program.

Cause and effect in occupational respiratory disease are very important, since such data help to determine the necessity and degree of worker protection and the type of medical surveillance necessary. For instance, cotton dust has been implicated in byssinosis but the mechanism is unclear. Some believe that byssinosis is an allergic reaction to the dust but no one has shown this to be the case. Estimates place the incidence of byssinosis at 6 percent of the textile mill work

Table 5: Agents Causing Transient and Permanent Respiratory Disorders

Agent	Disease
Acetic acid	Bronchopneumonia, pulmonary edema, catarrh, bronchitis
Allyl alcohol	Upper respiratory tract irritant
Ammonia	Airway irritation
Amyl alcohol	Respiratory tract irritant
Antimony	Lung effects
Asphalt fumes	Respiratory irritant
Benzene	Pulmonary edema
Benzoyl peroxide	Airway irritation
Beryllium	Sarcoidosis, pulmonary fibrosis
Boron trifluoride	Respiratory system effects
Bromine and hydrogen bromide	Upper respiratory irritant
Cadmium and its compounds	Severe pulmonary irritation, emphysema
Carbon dioxide	Respiratory system effects
Chlorine	Industrial bronchitis
Coal dust	Pneumoconiosis (black lung)
Cyanide and cyanide salts	Airway irritation
	Respiratory system effects
DBCP	Respiratory irritation
	Pulmonary congestion and edema
Ethylene dibromide	Respiratory system effects
Ethylene dichloride	Respiratory system effects
Fibrous glass	Airway irritation
Formaldehyde	Lung effects
Graphite dust	Pneumoconiosis
Hydrogen fluoride	Airway irritation
Hydrogen sulfide	Respiratory system effects
Mineral dust (silica, asbestos)	Pulmonary fibrosis
Nitriles	Respiratory system effects
Nitrogen oxides	Emphysema
Organic dusts, coffee, cotton, cottonseed	Byssinosis (brown lung disease)
Ozone	Emphysema, bronchitis
Phosgene	Airway effects
Refined petroleum solvent	Lung irritation
Simple amines	
Sodium hydroxide	Airway irritation
Sulfur dioxide	Reduction of pulmonary function, irritation
Sulfuric acid	Pulmonary irritation
Tetrachloroethylene	Respiratory system effects
Toluene diisocyanate	Asthma, respiratory tract irritation
Trimellitic anhydride	Asthma, hemorrhage, pneumonia
Vanadium	Lung effects
Xylene	Airway irritation

force. Workers in the yarn preparation area have an estimated incidence of 20 percent. However, industries with stringent medical screening and supervision and effective dust removal systems report an incidence of about 1 percent. A study conducted by Yale Medical School estimates that there are currently 35,000 people disabled and retired suffering from byssinosis, in addition to those whose disease has not progressed to the disabling stages and are still employed.

REPRODUCTIVE AND FETAL DISORDERS

Originally, since most industrial workers were male, efforts in controlling hazards concentrated on identifying substances that were either mutagenic or

Table 6: Hazardous Substances Affecting Reproductive Function

Substance	Suspected Effects	Exposure Limits
Benzene		
Carbaryl	Teratogen	Minimal during pregnancy
Carbon disulfide	Teratogen	Minimal during pregnancy
Carbon tetrachloride	Teratogen	Minimal during pregnancy
Chloroform	Teratogen	Minimal during pregnancy
Chloroprene	Teratogen	Minimal during pregnancy
DBCP	Sterility	
Dioxin		
Endrin	Congenital defects	Minimal during pregnancy
Ethylene dibromide	Mutagen	
Ethylene dichloride	Toxic	Minimal during lactation
Ethylene oxide	Sterility/mutagenicity	Male
Ethylene thiourea	Mutagen/teratogen	Minimal during pregnancy
Glycidyl ethers	Mutagen	
Herbicides, general		
Hexachlorophene	Suspected teratogen	Minimal during pregnancy
Lead	Birth defects	Minimal in females of child-bearing age
Mercury		
Pesticides, general		
Polychlorinated biphenyls	Toxic	Minimal during lactation
Tetrachloroethylene	Congenital abnormalities	Minimal during pregnancy
Waste anesthetic gases and vapors		Minimal during pregnancy

caused sterility in men. Lately, with more and more women employed by industry, the possibility of fetal damage in pregnant workers, and the deleterious effects on infants of nursing mothers, has created a new flurry of regulations and concern.

The problems are compounded by the lack of adequate data regarding the effects of chemicals on the reproductive system. NIOSH lists (see Table 6) several substances that are suspected of causing teratogenicity, mutagenicity, sterility, and other reproductive abnormalities. Also, two substances are listed as posing a threat to the infants of nursing mothers exposed to these substances.

Reproductive function hazards affect millions of workers in hundreds of different manufacturing processes. Although both men and women are at risk, the problem becomes even more serious when women of childbearing age or pregnant women are involved. Since 41 percent of the work force is female, the challenge to maintain fetal health is unquestionably one of the top priorities of occupational medicine.

Agents causing sterility in men include such chemicals as ethyl dibromide and such pesticides as Kepone and DBCP. Agents causing chromosomal damage in the exposed population and suspected of affecting the pregnancy outcome of spouses of affected workers include vinyl chloride, chloroprene, and benzene. Women exposed to anesthetic gases suffer decreased fertility and increased rate of spontaneous abortions and there is some evidence for a link between such exposure and an increase in infant birth defects.

Another major source of concern is low-level radiation. Although the mutagenic effects of radiation have been demonstrated in animals, the effects in the human are still not established.

CARDIOVASCULAR DISEASE

Cardiovascular disease is the most prevalent cause of death and disability. The cost of the loss of industrial output due to cardiovascular diseases is an estimated $8.1 billion annually. Also, it has been estimated that for every 1000 employees screened, a minimum of 100 individuals will have two or more coronary risk factors.

Cardiovascular disease appears to be more a factor of personal habits and genetic predisposition than of occupational exposure. However, one risk factor associated with cardiovascular disease, stress, is often generated by the work environment.

Other occupational hazards associated with heart disease include:

- toxic gases, when inhaled, may affect the electromechanical performance of muscle, particularly the myocardium,
- carbon monoxide and carbon disulfide are mutagenic and are suspected of playing an important role in the development of atherosclerosis,
- lead causes cardiotoxicity after long-term exposures.

Table 7: Agents Suspected of Causing Cardiovascular Disorders

Agents	Disorders
Antimony	Heart effects
Carbon black	Heart effects
Carbon disulfide	Mutagen—promotes atherosclerosis
Carbon monoxide	Mutagen—promotes atherosclerosis
Ethylene dibromide	Heart effects
Ethylene dichloride	Heart effects
Lead	Cardiotoxicity
Nitriles	Heart effects
Nitroglycerin	Circulatory system effects
Organotin compounds	
Tetrachloroethylene	

A list of industrial substances that produce cardiovascular disorders upon exposure are listed in Table 7.

OTHER DISORDERS CAUSED BY TOXIC AGENTS

Workplace toxins can affect virtually every organ system of the body, causing various health effects.

The most vulnerable body systems are those directly exposed to workplace hazards, such as skin and the eyes. Numerous substances are toxic to the skin and eyes, as listed in Table 3. Often skin disorders caused by toxic substances mimic those naturally occurring among the nonexposed population and present a challenge to the occupational physician. Eye irritation is also common but exposure to some substances can cause permanent damage or blindness.

Numerous workplace hazards can also cause neurological disorders, depending on the severity and duration of exposure. Table 8 lists some of these agents. Symptoms upon exposure range from headache and nausea to narcosis and seizures and sometimes death.

Workplace stress may also cause psychological and behavioral aberrations that could endanger the health of the affected worker as well as his co-workers.

Other organs vulnerable to toxic substances are the liver and the kidneys, which are the organs responsible for the detoxification and excretion of hazardous substances. Tables 9 and 10 list major industrial agents suspected of causing liver and kidney disorders.

Early diagnosis of detrimental effects to the kidneys and liver is difficult because symptoms do not appear until significant damage occurs.

Table 8: Agents Causing Central Nervous System Disorders

Agent	Effect
Acetates	CNS depression
Acetylene	Asphyxiation
Acrylamide	CNS effects
Alkanes	CNS effects
Alcohols	CNS depression
Arsine	Cellular toxins
Arsenic	CNS disorders
Carbaryl	CNS effects
Carbon disulfide	Cellular toxins
Carbon monoxide	Oxygen deprivation
Chloroform	CNS effects
Dinitro-ortho-cresol	CNS effects
Ethers	CNS depression
Ethylene dibromide	CNS damage
Ethylene dichloride	CNS effects
Halogenated hydrocarbons	CNS depression
Hydrogen cyanide	Cellular toxins
Hydrogen sulfide	Cellular toxins
Kepone	CNS damage
Ketones	
Lead	CNS disorders
Malathion	Nervous system effects
Manganese	CNS disorders
Mercury	CNS disorders
Methyl parathion	CNS effects
Methylene chloride	CNS effects
Nitriles	CNS effects
Organotin compounds	CNS effects
Parathion	CNS effects
Phenol	CNS effects
Pesticides, general	CNS disorders
Stilbene	Cellular toxins
Styrene	CNS depression
1, 1, 2, 2-Tetrachloroethane	CNS effects
Tetrachloroethylene	CNS effects
Thiols	CNS effects
Toluene	CNS depression
1, 1, 1, -Trichloroethane	CNS effects
Trichloroethylene	CNS depression
Xylene	CNS depression

Table 9: Agents that May Cause Liver Damage

Acetonitrile	Ethylene dichloride
Acrylonitrile	Ethyl silicate
Allyl chloride	Hydrazine
Antimony	Ketones
Arsine	Manganese
Benzene	Methyl alcohol
Beryllium	Methyl chloride
Bismuth	Naphthalene
Bromoform	Nitriles
Cadmium	Nitrobenzene
Carbon tetrabromide	Organotin
Carbon tetrachloride	Phenol
Chloroprene	Phenylhydrazine
Chloroform	Polychlorinated biphenyls
Cresol	Propylene dichloride
DBCP	Pyridine
DDT	Selenium
Dimethyl sulfate	Styrene
Dinitrophenol	1, 1, 2, 2-Tetrachloroethane
Dioxane	Tetrachloroethylene
Epichlorohydrin	Toluene
Ethyl alcohol	1, 1, 1, -Trichloroethane
Ethylene bromide	Trichloroethylene
Ethylene chlorohydrin (beta-chloroethanol)	Yellow phosphorus

Table 10: Agents that May Cause Kidney Disease

Acute carbon monoxide poisoning	Fluoride
Allyl chloride	Heat stroke
Arsenic	Ketones
Arsine	Lead
Bismuth	Mercury
Cadmium	Nitriles
Carbon disulfide	Oxalic acid
Carbon tetrachloride	Phenol
Chromium	Tartrates
Chronic exposure to heat	1, 1, 2, 2-Tetrachloroethane
DBCP	Uranium
Dioxane	Vibration
Ethylene glycol	

5
Techniques in Identifying Harmful Environments

The ideal approach in the identification of a harmful environment is pretesting of all substances present in the environment for toxicity and elimination of those that appear harmful. This of course, may be difficult to do. Presently, there are 15,000 chemicals manufactured in the United States and there are thousands of processes utilizing them in various combinations. Pretoxicity testing will probably identify those that are either highly toxic in a small dose or carcinogenic in low concentrations over a period of time. But other hazardous possibilities, such as toxicity due to a combination of substances that are individually innocuous, or health effects that manifest themselves years after the initial exposure, are difficult to identify. Also, in many cases, protective devices and ambient air monitoring might be inadequate to protect the worker over long-term exposure. Finally, genetic predisposition and an individual's life style could be critical in assessing the risks of a certain manufacturing environment on such a worker.

Therefore, although stricter requirements in pretesting of industrial substances are in the works and tough standards have been promulgated regarding worker exposure to hazardous environments, the role of occupational medicine continues to become more and more important and medical techniques will play a very crucial role in the industrial health area.

Undoubtedly, however, knowledge of the harmful effects of industrial substances will become more and more necessary to safeguard the health of the workforce. Two techniques, toxicology and epidemiology, are the most important methods available today to assess the potential harm of environmental and occupational hazards on the health of the general population and the workforce.

TOXICOLOGY

Toxicology is a method of identifying hazardous materials in the work environment, establishing their short- and long-term effects on animals and therefore also potentially on human beings, and identifying and measuring their presence in man after exposure to known toxic substances.

The Department of Health and Human Sciences (DHHS) has initiated the National Toxicology Program to coordinate the research on toxic substances, by combining the efforts of four federal agencies that study such substances. The new program includes the following agencies: NCI, FDA, NIEHS, NIOSH.

The task of the program is to test some of the chemicals not fully tested for safety as yet. Out of about 70,000 chemicals in use, fewer than 2500 have been tested at all for carcinogenicity. Current testing capability is about 500 agents annually, which is expected to be boosted significantly by the creation of this new program. Other toxic effects of substances under investigation, in addition to carcinogenicity, are also to be established by the program. First year budget is estimated at about $40 million.

Toxicology is becoming big business. Manufacturers, especially those in the vulnerable industries, such as chemical and food production, are creating a comprehensive in-house capability to pretest or monitor substances manufactured at their plants to identify potential hazards before they evolve into an economic or health catastrophe.

Proctor & Gamble, for instance, operates one of the nation's largest toxicology laboratories employing more than 200 scientists. Other manufacturers, such as Dow Chemical, Stauffer Chemical, Monsanto, E.I. DuPont de Nemours, and Litton Industries, either currently run or are planning to run their own toxicology laboratories, often offering their services to outside clients. Also, leading companies in the chemical industry have created the Institute of Toxicology, a $12 million facility located in Research Triangle Park, North Carolina.

All in all, there are about 200 independent toxicology laboratories in the United States, but fewer than 50 are of any size. It is estimated that the total revenue of this industry exceeds $500 million and is growing at 25 percent annually.

The passage of TOSCA presently administered by the EPA has intensified the need for better approaches to toxicity evaluations. During the Carter era toxicity testing often resulted in the banning of certain substances or in the introduction of exposure and control requirements for others; industry balked on occasion at the testing procedures used. The most popular technique of toxicity testing is the maximum tolerated dose (MTD) approach. This method relies on exposing animals to huge doses of the suspected substance and, if toxic, assume that it would also affect man in a similar way. Another test, with many limitations, is one devised by Dr. Ames. It uses a special strain of Salmonella bacteria that mutate rapidly when exposed to carcinogens. New tests, such as those using human cells, are expected to introduce refinements that would produce more conclusive results.

A test with some promise is the *B. subtilis* Comptest devised by Dr. Ronald Yasbin, which takes advantage of a genetic repair mechanism in the DNA of the bacterium. An unknown factor activated by carcinogens triggers this repair mechanism and also triggers the quiescent viruses within the cell, which multiply rapidly and kill the host cell. The speed and degree of cell death indicate the carcinogenicity of the substance under investigation.

Expansion of life-sciences facilities could reach 50 percent per year, but staffing is a real problem because of a shortage of trained personnel.

EPIDEMIOLOGY

Epidemiology plays a very important role in the identification of environmental hazards and their effects on human beings. Since much of toxicological research is performed on animals, the findings are oftentimes criticized when they are presented as applying equally to the human being. Epidemiology can be used to verify such findings by studying certain population groups that have been exposed to the hazard under consideration for known amounts of time and degree of exposure. Epidemiological research was difficult to perform in the past because workers' medical records were hopelessly incomplete. The new regulatory environment, however, with strict guidelines regarding occupational exposure and medical surveillance will provide this science with all the necessary data to produce accurate information on the effects of workplace agents on employee health.

Epidemiologists and statisticians are currently developing models and techniques to study several difficult problems associated with environmental and human interactions, such as multiple cause mortality, disease linkage, and genetic predisposition, to define the risk for given population groups.

Epidemiology is most important in the identification of carcinogens, mutagens, and teratogens in the environment in general and in the workplace in particular. Since the identification of substances causing cancers in the human is an inexact science, epidemiological evidence can confirm laboratory findings that are most often derived from animal experimentation. For instance, although there is laboratory evidence that links smoking to cancer, it is the epidemiological proof that the two are connected that has enabled scientists to arrive at a health-related conclusion.

Epidemiology is uniquely suited for identifying hazardous environments leading to the diseases of the modern age. Unlike those of the past, these disorders do not have a single cause that can be easily identified and isolated but are caused by many factors of different importance and gravity. Life-science evaluations have had limited success in identifying these factors, in spite of the enormous amount of funds provided for research. Epidemiology currently appears to have a better chance at isolating some of the causes of occupationally induced diseases.

As a result of the wider application of epidemiology in human disease, there is an increasing demand for trained professionals in this field. A recent survey of research organizations conducted at UCLA[19] serves to underscore the fact that many positions for epidemiologists at the masters and doctoral level remain unfilled today. If the demand in institutions is so great, it can be easily surmised that industry will also be seeking such professionals in increasing numbers, so that it can remain abreast of any research that reflects upon certain occupations or manufacturing processes.

6
Medical Surveillance

In-house medical surveillance is an expensive undertaking for industry, but it is gradually becoming both necessary and desirable. Naturally, the first to adopt some kind of in-plant capability to monitor employees' health status was the large corporation. Today, it is safe to say that most large corporations maintain some form of in-plant medical or health-care personnel. However, these departments cover only 25 percent of the total work force and do not represent the realities of the status of occupational medicine in the United States. Smaller companies are following suit, albeit slowly and cautiously. For instance, in 1977, according to labor statistics, the most hazardous places to work were the small companies with fewer than 25 employees. Such establishments cannot afford the luxury of in-house medical surveillance.

Naturally, there are many different ways to assure that employees receive adequate medical attention. The most desirable approach is to maintain a medically trained staff at the site. Another is to retain the services of an outside physician, private clinic, or hospital knowledgeable in industrial medicine to provide services on a part-time or as needed basis.

Whatever the mode of medical surveillance, demand by industry will increase rapidly in the future. Also, the responsibilities and tasks of the health professionals associated with occupational medicine will increase in scope and sophistication, requiring more training, better education, and more stringent certification, and also offering such professionals a brighter occupational and financial future.

The respondents to the F&S survey were overwhelmingly in support of a regular screening regimen for industrial workers. Approximately 70 percent answered positively and only 6.4 percent were plainly against it. The remainder of the respondents provided some qualifications, such as:

for hazardous occupations only and depending on job exposure,
only if individuals assume responsibility for their own health,
only in few instances,
baseline only,
only based on age and occupational history,
only if individuals have chronic problems,
desirable but not necessary,
conventional screening is questionable as a promoter of health,
and
not as a protective measure but only to measure effectiveness of environmental controls.

Those who answered negatively suggested that other methods, such as health education, might be more effective. Those who answered positively often qualified their statements by limiting screening to those in hazardous occupations and those over critical ages. Overall, however, the consensus is that periodic medical screening is considered helpful and even necessary within certain industries and certain employee groups.

Additionally, about 63 percent of the respondents believe that a periodic medical examination program would be mandated by law and only about 11 percent thought that such a law was not imminent. Many gave tongue-in-cheek answers but many believed the law was already here, quoting selected OSHA standards. Some, however, volunteered comments that illustrate the range of views about the issue. A selected sample of these comments follows:

If the screening program is legislated it would be part of a total federal socialized medical program.
The advent of a law to require medical screening will become a reality if businessmen/manufacturers do not show better compliance with certain regulations.
Some basic screening on all employees should be done (vision, hearing, blood tests).
Probably the government will require medical screening in the future but we offer it now regardless as we can do a better job at lower cost than that mandated by any government sponsored program.
First we must solve the problem of job tenure and availability of alternate employment for those found medically unfit.
Each occupation will have a certain testing regimen.
Mandatory medical screening interferes with the rights of the individual.

Private industry should not bear the burden of cost. Such a program can be forced in industry only if it is subsidized by the government. Even if required, it cannot be currently implemented.

OCCUPATIONAL MEDICINE AND HEALTH PROFESSIONALS

Naturally, the core of an occupational medicine program is the physician, preferably a specialist. In the past, due to the lack of interest in this area, medical school trained specialists were rare. Today, this is changing rapidly as more and more medical schools create occupational medicine departments. Other health professionals associated with occupational medicine are nurses, public health specialists, and industrial hygienists. Their role in industry is:

to define and record work-related deaths, injuries, and illnesses
to alert employers to unsuspected hazards present in the manufacturing process,
to provide preemployment examinations and periodic examinations as needed
to provide screening, diagnosis, and treatment of work-related diseases and injuries,
to assess impairment of injured or convalescent employees returning to work, and, in some instances,
to design and carry out epidemiological studies and other research projects.

In 1977 NIOSH undertook a study to determine the existing occupational safety and health force and to develop a manpower forecasting model to estimate future requirements in this field.[43] The results of the study are presented in Table 11. These results, however, appear to have grossly underestimated the available professional resources in this area, which becomes apparent from our findings presented in this section.

The professional and employment status of those responding to the F&S direct mail survey is given in Table 12. As expected, the majority of the respondents are physicians, representing 66.4 percent of the total. The next largest group are nurses with 23.6 percent of the total. Hygienists make up a very small portion of the total.

Physicians

Compliance with safety and health regulations created a new physician specialty, i.e., occupational medicine. According to a definition put forth by the American Medical Association "occupational medicine means that branch of medicine practiced by physicians in meeting medical problems and needs within a program, provided usually by management, to deal constructively with the health of employees in relation to their job."

Table 11: Estimated 1977 National Occupational Safety and Health Work Force by Industry and Basic Area

Industry	Safety	Radiation	Industrial Hygiene	Fire Protection	General	Medical	Not Classified	Total†
Mining	1,170	50	200	90	750	10	60	2,330
Construction	2,350	40	0	30	380	100	190	3,080
Manufacturing	16,440	180	1,130	1,770	8,380	7,320	2,450	37,670
Transportation, communication, and utilities	4,261	0	150	250	1,580	140	850	7,230
Trades, services, and non-OSH Government	3,970	440	200	1,910	3,750	2,190	1,270	13,720
Insurance	4,330	0	190	810	3,350	0	850	9,520
OSH-related state government	1,910	0	1,120	0	460	20	520	4,020
Federal	2,840	660	1,820	90	1,360	220	290	7,270
Total†	37,260	1,370	4,810	4,950	19,990	9,990	6,490	84,850

*Basic area refers to the task of the work force that occupies more than 50% of his or her professional time.
†Totals may not add due to rounding.
SOURCE: *A Nationwide Survey of the Occupational Safety and Health Work Force*, NIOSH, 1978.

Table 12. Survey Respondents by Professional and Employment Status

Professional Status*†	No. of Respondents	% of Total	Employment Status				
			Full Time	% of Total	Part Time	% of Total	N/A	% of Total

Professional Status*†	No. of Respondents	% of Total	Full Time	% of Total	Part Time	% of Total	N/A	% of Total
Physician	284	66.4	176	61.9	81	28.5	27	9.6
Nurse	101	23.6	85	84.4	12	11.8	4	3.8
Industrial hygienist	30	7	14	46.7	9	30	7	23.3
Other	13	3	9	69.2	—	—	4	30.8
Total	428	100	284	66.4	102	23.8	42	9.8

*Titles included:

Physicians: Medical Director; Health Services Director; Plant Physician; Chief, Occupational Medicine; Vice President; Staff Physician; Director of Occupational Health; Area Medical Director; Regional Medical Director; Chief Surgeon; Corporate Medical Director; Medical Officer; Associate Medical Director; Consultant; Director of Industrial Health; Medical Supervisor; Regional Flight Surgeon; Medical Advisor; Medical Group Leader; Director, Health Services; Psychiatrist; Director of Public Health.

Nurses: Supervisor, Medical Services; Technician; Associate Director; Director of Safety and the Environment; Occupational Health Nurse; Head Nurse; Chief Nurse; Manager, Employee Health Service; Plant Nurse; Corporate Nurse; Director of Nurses; Supervisor, Safety and Health Training; Site Nurse; Medical Supervisor, Director of Health Services, Manager, Nursing Services; Coordinator, Employee Medical Services.

Industrial Hygienists: VP, Engineering; Safety and Security Supervisor; Manager, Industrial Hygiene; Manager, Environmental Compliance; Safety Director; Sr. Health Consultant; VP, Safety Services; Assistant Manager of Safety; Director, Occupational Health and Safety.

Other: Safety Director; Loss Control Manager; Manager, Safety and Health; Personnel Administrator; Director, Product Stewardship; Vice President, Safety and Health; Director of Benefits and Personnel Services; Emergency Medical Technician; Physician Associate; Professor, Community Medicine; Safety Director.

†Does not include service providers and consultants.

The NIOSH Study[43] estimates that there were 1010 occupational physicians employed by industry and the federal government on a full or part time basis in 1976. Nearly 62 percent of these physicians were full-time employees. This estimate is too low unless it is interpreted as the total number of physicians employed by industry directly rather than hired for special consultations only or as needed. The American Occupational Medical Association has 4000 members directly involved in occupational medicine. Some are practicing abroad, but the majority concentrate their practice in occupational medicine in the United States. Also the American Board of Preventive Medicine has, to date, certified 800 physicians as occupational medicine specialists. Estimates of the number of physicians who practice occupational medicine as part of their medical practice range from 12,000 to 20,000.

As long ago as 1969, a study prepared by the AMA, using the data given in the membership roster of the Industrial Medical Association, identified 2438 physicians employed by industry or by institutions. at least 1923 were employed directly by industry. These data represent the state of affairs even before OSHA was created, and it is safe to assume that the numbers of physicians working with industry has increased significantly since 1970.

The demand for occupational specialists will continue to be strong in the future, as industry is gearing up to meet the regulatory demands in the area of employee safety and health. Opportunities for specially trained physicians abound, in industry, in health care institutes, in academia, and in independent private practice. Some of the positions available in industry are presented in Table 12. Other employment choices include:

Private or group practice in occupational medicine providing services to industry under contract.
Hospital staff positions in occupational medicine departments.
Teaching positions in the many newly created occupational medicine programs.
Research in epidemiology and preventive medicine.
Government positions in research and regulation.

Full-time industrial physicians command handsome compensation, with starting salaries estimated at the $45,000 to $50,000 levels.

It is estimated that there is a shortage of 5000 to 6000 physicians specifically trained and certified in occupational medicine.

Nurses

Nurses represent the most widely employed health professionals in the industrial setting. The NIOSH survey[43] estimates that in 1977 there were 8980 nurses employed by industry, the majority (89 percent) in full-time positions. Of these 71.3 percent are registered nurses (RN). The next largest group is represented by the licensed practical nurses (LPN), at 15.9 percent of the total. Another NIOSH study[42] placed the number of RN and LPN employed by the manufacturing industries alone at 12.494 and 1286, respectively.

The occupational health nurse is often the only health professional employed on a full-time basis by industry, especially in small plants. The traditional role of the industrial nurse is to provide on-site first aid. However, as regulatory developments placed more and more emphasis on the health rather than only the safety of the worker, the nurses' role has expanded to include coordinations of the plants' health and safety program.

Average starting salaries are estimated at $13-14,000.

Approximately 24 percent of the respondents to our survey were nurses. The majority were RNs and were a part of an established in-house medical department.

It is expected that occupational nurses will play an increasingly major role in this field as the requirements for medical surveillance expand to cover more and more industries and as the cost of such surveillance becomes more and more burdensome for many smaller firms. For instance, in its cotton dust standard, OSHA suggests that if trained nurses perform the pulmonary function testing required a company can save nearly 12 percent of the cost of paying an outside service.

Industrial Hygienists

Industrial hygienists represent the second largest group of professionals involved in an important way with employee health. The NIOSH study[43] estimates that in 1977 there were approximately 4810 industrial hygienists employed by industry and government in occupational safety and health positions. Approximately 89 percent of industrial hygienists held full-time positions. Most had a B.S. degree and such a degree was a requirement for employment in 75 percent of the cases.

Average beginning salaries were in the range of $13-14,000.

Only 7 percent of the respondents to our survey were industrial hygienists, illustrating the fact that in cases of established medical departments the industrial hygienist's role is more in ensuring a healthful working environment rather than assuming medical care responsibility.

MEDICAL SURVEILLANCE TECHNIQUES

Medical surveillance varies from industry to industry and plant to plant. There are steps that must be taken with all workers, as well as specific requirements that relate only to segments of the working population. The form of medical surveillance adopted at each facility is based on the working environment. Workers performing tasks associated with less hazardous processes have less need for aggressive medical surveillance than those engaged in activities carrying a higher potential health risk.

Generally, all industries with even the rudiments of an occupational health program offer a preplacement examination or screening to all incoming employees. Also companies provide medical services for job-related accidents or health problems. However, to date, there are no strict regulations regarding the degree of medical surveillance necessary to ensure employee safety from occupationally induced diseases. All this is expected to change as it is realized that adherence to regulations regarding the work environment are not sufficient to prevent occupational illness and an aggressive medical surveillance is often necessary to identify early symptoms of disease. Often environmental monitoring alone leads to a false sense of security and prevents early diagnosis of health problems associated with the type of work performed. An aggressive medical surveillance program consists of the following services:

Preplacement Examination. The standard preplacement examination includes the following:

personal and family medical history,
occupational history,
physical examination and those laboratory tests deemed appropriate, and
special screening for preconditions that would render employment in a certain area highly hazardous.

Preplacement examinations insure that an individual is placed in the appropriate job regarding the physical demands and risks of the work and the employee's health status.

OSHA recommends that the medical examination includes the personal and family occupational history of the employee, including genetic and environmental factors.

Taking a comprehensive medical history is a requirement in all surveillance programs recommended by OSHA and NIOSH. Such a record should contain:

a complete medical history, including special emphasis on organ system at risk, depending on the type of the exposure hazard,
a complete occupational history,
a record of any drugs taken by the worker, and
a record of any personal habits (smoking, drinking, poor nutrition) that could introduce additional risk factors unrelated to the work environment.

Industries that engage in operations that expose their workers to OSHA-regulated substances also include the following medical surveillance programs in their health screening regimen:

Pretoxic Indicators. These tests are performed in hazardous industries before clinical findings become apparent. Such tests must be easily performed, must be fast, cheap, and reproducible, such as a free erythrocyte protoporphyrin test for lead.

Periodic Examinations. The periodicity of medical screening or examination is currently dependent on employer policies. Workers employed in hazardous jobs are likely to be examined more frequently, whereas those engaging in safer activities might not be examined at all. Periodic examinations could be general physical screening procedures or highly targeted tests specifically to identify disorders relating to the type of the work environment to which an employee is exposed. OSHA is contemplating making periodic medical examinations mandatory.

Periodic examinations can insure an employee's health throughout his or her working career. Such examinations also serve to pinpoint early phases of occupational diseases.

Episodic Examinations. Episodic examinations are performed when a worker has a specific complaint or when it is believed that a certain group of workers has been exposed to dangerous levels of toxic or disease-producing contaminants. Episodic examinations might involve a one-time visit to a physician or could involve a continuous medical surveillance program.

Medical surveillance programs in industries with workers exposed to OSHA-regulated substances vary according to the type of substances encountered in the workplace and their toxicity.

Workplace hazards can be classified into three separate categories regarding medical surveillance requirements:

Low Potential (Highly Toxic Effects at Exposure). Highly toxic sunstances are the easiest to deal with when it comes to medical monitoring requirements. Such substances as acetone, camphor, and acetic acid cause acute toxicity, but their chronic low-grade effects are minimal. The monitoring of workers handling such materials consists of taking a medical history and screening for preconditions at the time of employment. Thereafter, only those with preconditions (estimated at 10 percent of the total workforce) need to have a physical examination.

Medium Potential (Cumulative Effects). These agents pose a medical surveillance challenge and require an aggressive worker monitoring program. Most of the developments in occupationsl medicine have been concentrated in devising screening methods to protect workers from hazards that act on a cumulative principle or have long latent periods.

Least Toxic Substances. Workers handling such substances need not be monitored, since any toxic effects from these agents are reversible.

Initially, OSHA developed separate standards for each major hazard, especially if found to be carcinogenic. Such individual standards are discussed in the sections of this study describing the hazardous substances. The current philosophy, however, is to develop a blanket medical surveillance program that would apply generally to each category of toxins, as discussed in chapter 3.

All medical examinations are free and conducted during regular working hours. Industry must keep records of all such examinations, treatment given, and any steps taken toward amelioration of exposure.

Another type of medical surveillance, almost always assumed by a company, without any government involvement, is the executive health screening program currently used by numerous corporations. These programs are offered selectively to certain company personnel and vary in depth, depending on the subject's age and general health.

Executive examinations are often criticized as ineffective because on a statistical basis they detect small numbers of serious organic diseases. However, they provide a periodic health assessment for the employee and have a preventive function, that is, executives are placed on a diet if cholesterol levels appear ominous, are advised to stop smoking, are counseled regarding exercise, and often are helped with mental problems.

Most executive screening programs are age-related, being offered to employees who are 40 years of age or older. There are several theories as to the type of screening most appropriate, but almost always it offers an EKG examination, blood chemistry and hematology test, and hearing and vision tests. Some programs have also included stress testing and proctoscopy as part of the regimen for men and breast examination and Pap smears for women. With the exception of the Pap smear, these tests have been considered unnecessary, since they rarely result in early diagnosis, when disease prognosis is favorable. For instance, stress testing of asymptomatic individuals results in too many false positives and proctoscopy, an uncomfortable procedure, rarely detects early disorders in asymptomatic individuals.

MEDICAL RECORD KEEPING REQUIREMENTS

Maintenance of complete and accurate medical records is a requirement in all industries. OSHA requires that employers keep injury and illness records for each establishment. An establishment is defined as a "single physical location where business is conducted or where services are performed." An employer whose employees work in dispersed locations must keep his or her records at the place where the employees report for work. In some situations, employees do not report to work at the same place each day, in which case, records must be kept at the place from which they are paid or at the base from which they operate.

There are two record-keeping forms that must be maintained on a calendar year basis. They are not sent to OSHA, but rather they are kept at the establishment and made available for OSHA inspection for a period of five years following the end of the year recorded. These forms are:

OSHA No. 101 Supplementary Records: Each recordable injury or illness must be recorded in detail within six working days from the time the employer learns of it. Substitutes for the form, such as insurance or workers' compensation forms, may be used if they contain all the information required.

OSHA No. 200 Log and Summary of Occupational Injuries and Illnesses: Each recordable occupational injury or illness also must be logged on this form within six working days from the time the employer learns of it. Recorded information will include: the date of each injury or onset of illness, the employee's name and occupation, the department in which he or she works, the nature of the injury or illness, the type of illness (where applicable), the number of lost workdays, and whether a termination or transfer was required. The employer may choose not to utilize OSHA No. 200; however, any private equivalent must contain the same information in a form as complete and as easily understood. Within one month after the close of the year, the employer must compile a job injury and illness summary, based on the information in the log, and post the summary in the establishment for no less than 30 days.

In addition to safety and health standards and record-keeping duties, employers are responsible for keeping their employees informed about OSHA and about the various safety and health matters with which they are involved. OSHA requires that each employer post certain materials at a prominent location in the workplace. These include:

Job Safety and Health Protection (workplace poster, OSHA 2203), informing employees of their rights and responsibilities under the Occupational Safety and Health Act. Besides displaying the workplace poster, the employer must make copies of the Act and copies of OSHA rules and regulations relevant to the workplace available to employees upon request.

Summaries of petitions for variances from standards of record-keeping procedures.

Copies of OSHA citations for violations of standards. These must remain posted for three days, or until the violations are abated, whichever is longer.

Summary of Occupational Injuries and Illnesses (OSHA No. 200), which must be posted within one month of the close of the year, and remain posted for at least 30 days.

Occasionally, OSHA standards or NIOSH research activities will require an employer to measure and record employee exposure to potentially harmful substances. All employees have the right (in person or through their authorized representative) to be present during the measuring and to examine the records kept of the results.

Each employee or former employee has the right to see his or her own examination records and must be told by the employer if the exposure to hazardous substances has exceeded the levels set by OSHA. The employee must also be told what corrective measures, if any, are being taken.

In addition OSHA requires that an employer preserve all records regarding worker exposure to dangerous levels of hazardous substances and the results of job-related examinations.

The maintenance of comprehensive employee health records should provide an excellent means of monitoring the incidence and prevalence of occupationally induced diseases. It is an invaluable epidemiological tool that could in the long term exclusively establish the degree of risk inherent in every industrial process based on many worker variables, such as age, personal habits, and genetic predisposition. This is an exciting research tool with undisputed long-term benefits.

However, record keeping has many drawbacks. Aside from being costly to the employer it is also open to abuse regarding the employees right to privacy. As OSHA ponders its final regulations in the area of employee medical records, the debate over access to such records rages in many quarters. The Privacy Protection Study Commission, convened in 1974, recommends that the individual has the right of access to his records. OSHA has issued rules that require the employer to provide worker access to the "log and summary of occupational illnesses and injuries," which until recently was only available to federal and state officials. The individual would have the right of access for up to five years after termination.

Physicians, as expected, object to the indiscriminate access of patients to their own records for fear of unjustified law suits and to avoid administrative costs that overburden the system. However, access to the health records by well-informed patients should not create such a problem and the basic rationale behind the access concept is to force the industrial physician to be completely frank with the employee. Also, it has been found that a well-informed patient is better equipped to deal with his medical problem.

Many would label the health-record access controversy "phony" issue, since in the past many third parties, such as top management and insurers, had access to records denied to the employee or his representative union. A reasonable alternative to the preservation of the right to privacy is to provide all records to federal agencies after unrelated personal data and patient identification are removed.

Another alternative to the medical record access problem is to categorize medical records and allow access to different categories within the medical record to each interested party, that is, patient, employer, and government, and therefore prevent the total compromise of confidentiality.

Another issue cropping up in this area is malpractice. Access to records can result in suits directly brought against the attending physician if he is an independent provider, not employed by the company requesting the testing. The fact that in occupational medicine the physician examines the patient in behalf of a third party, that is, the employer or the insurer, alters the doctor-patient relationship irrevocably and obscures the doctor's responsibility toward the person he has examined. The occupational or primary care physician hired by the company usually performs preemployment examinations and sometimes screens employees working with hazardous materials. Often the private physician is ill-equipped to perform esoteric assessments and if wrong he alone is liable. The expected increase in the number of specialists in occupational medicine should solve this problem.

MULTIPHASIC SCREENING—PREVENTIVE MEDICINE CONCEPTS

Preventive medicine is a new concept unproved and much criticized as ineffective. It has evolved as a result of technology that has created techniques to look into the body through its numerous windows without disturbing its integrity to any great extent. X-rays, body fluid tests, radioisotope procedures, vision and auditory tests, ultrasound, and blood pressure measuring devices have all contributed to the popularity of the multiphasic examination, a highly mechanized and highly standardized medical evaluation undertaken to identify early warnings of impending disease.

Although preventive medicine is widely considered a sound practice, it is nevertheless practiced on a very limited scale. Interestingly, industry is the most active participant in the field of multiphasic screening of asymptomatic individuals for the purpose of prevention of disease. Although laws requiring medical screening of employees are a new development, many industries have been screening their employees, offering a limited and highly targeted evaluation program, for several decades.

Currently, preventive medicine is undergoing close scrutiny by the medical profession, the government, and the consumer. If demonstrated to be of real value, the consumer will demand it, the government will require it, and the physician would have to be prepared to offer it. The first group of physicians that are specifically trained in preventive medicine are the occupational specialists.

Respondents to the F&S survey overwhelmingly agreed (88%) that preventive medicine is a workable concept within their area of endeavor. Some of the comments contributed by the respondents were as follows:

> Helpful programs include lectures, audiovisual aids, consultation on alcoholism, lungs and smoking.

Success depends on employee motivation, attitude, and cooperation.
Preventive medicine is economically necessary; cheaper in the long run.
Currently the climate is nonprofessional where materialistic goals prevail.
Employees do not respond unless preventive measures are enforced.
Management must be convinced; a dialogue is necessary.
Industry-sponsored programs offer the opportunity to provide health services and health education to those who may not receive such services anywhere else.
Management is just beginning to be aware of the benefits of a preventive medicine program.
Preventive medicine applications have a wide potential; little has been done in the past in this area.
Preventive medicine evaluations are not paid for by insurance.
Currently there are insufficient resources and support to implement such a program.
Low cost and demonstrable cost benefit are the keys to the acceptability of such a program.
Preventive medicine is a workable concept but currently it is not working too well.
Preventive medicine is encouraged and accepted by many companies but this reflects not the rule but the exception.
Preventive medicine through serological review and the use of immunological technology would be desirable.

Medical screening is only applicable for certain types of disorders that have the following attributes:

the disease has grave consequences, i.e., it is a serious health problem,
the prognosis of the course of the disorder is favorable when discovered in its early stages, and
the detection of early manifestations of the disease is possible via currently available testing methods.

The tests proposed must have high specificity and sensitivity and be inexpensive and cause minimal patient discomfort.

The type of medical screening performed also depends on the goals of the program. Although such programs are well-defined for employees exposed to OSHA-regulated substances, guidelines regarding screening the general population are ill-defined. An attempt has been made to design a lifetime health-monitoring system[8,45] that defines a testing regimen for certain age groups. Generally these programs are difficult to implement within the populace at large but the industrial setting presents an ideal forum to test the theories of preventive medicine. Within a few years the experience in this field will be a critical factor in deciding the future of preventive medicine.

7
Regulation, Legislation, and Research

As a field, occupational medicine brings together diverse interests: government, industry, consumer and professional groups, the workers whose health is being protected, and their unions, where they exist. Efforts to control risks to employee health and the technologies employed to achieve these ends are determined by these different interests.

As the single most powerful influence among these groups, the federal government has participated in every aspect of the development of the field of occupational medicine. The government plays a leading role by setting new rules for industry, performing research, uncovering new health hazards, and aiding firms to comply with its regulations. To a large extent, the scope and size of occupational medicine are determined by the kind and level of participation of the federal government in it. While the role of the government in the field has encountered resistance, especially of late, its central place in the field is assured; if anything, its position will get stronger rather than weaker.

The role of other interests has been less central or visible. Unions defend the rights of their members to an environment free from health risks, but have not always concurred with the positions taken by the government. Often these cases have brought to the surface fear of plant closures and lay-offs because of employers' inability or refusal to invest in improving the work environment. Some unions have been vocal; others, though they may have started their own organizations to grapple with the issues raised, have remained quiescent.

At first, private industry did little or nothing and hoped that interest in and government regulation of occupation health would both lapse. More recently, it has begun to take matters seriously and has found that it is not an altogether bad thing. Some large corporations, by relying upon their well-financed in-house medical departments, have experienced declining rates of absenteeism and reductions in high workmen's compensation claims while discovering that productivity has improved. It appears that many large corporations have considered providing some type of health screening for their employees.

These trends suggest that occupational medicine will grow as a field, and new technology associated with it will also gain in importance.

FEDERAL GOVERNMENT

The role of the government is omnipresent. New legislation expands the power of federal agencies and increases the demand for occupational medical services. More elaborate and far-reaching regulations increase the depth and sophistication of industrial health care departments. Finally, special financial and educational aid programs help small and medium-sized companies meet the health and safety requirements stipulated by law.

Research funded by federal monies increases our knowledge of potential hazards and their effects. Other programs, including manpower training, education, and funding of specialized environmental research centers, increase the human and scientific resources able to deal with environmental and occupational health matters.

Public awareness of the dangers of environmental pollution and the proliferation of man-made toxic and carcinogenic substances has also served to increase the participation of the federal government. Congress has actively sought to legislate strict measures for the protection of both the general population and workers at risk and has maintained oversight on all current measures to encourage enforcement of the law. A summary of the nature and scope of the federal government's involvement in the field of occupational health follows.

Federally Sponsored Research Programs

Thirteen federal agencies (see Table 13) report receiving funds for environmental health research. Total funding for research in 1979 was estimated at $584.4 million, up 5 percent from 1978. Areas of major concern include: determining the effects of air pollution on the general population, assessing the deleterious consequences of ingesting food additives, and estimating the potential damage to the environment caused by radiation. Most agencies, however, have also launched an extensive effort to address the health problems encountered in the workplace.

DHHS supplies most of the federal funds for research on occupational health; within the department the largest research entity is the National Institutes of Health (NIH). Several agencies within the NIH conduct research on different aspects of the relationship between workplace hazards and disease: NIEHS, NCI, NHLBI, the National Institute of General Medical Sciences (NIGMS), the National Institute of Neurological and Communicative Disorders and Stroke

(NINCDS), the National Institute of Allergy and Infectious Diseases (NIAID), the National Eye Institute (NEI), the National Institute of Arthritis, Diabetes, and Digestive and Kidney Diseases (NIADDKD), and the National Library of Medicine.

The CDC, established within the DHHS, also serves a major function in research on occupational health risks, largely because it is the parent agency for NIOSH. NIOSH concentrates exclusively on research to determine the effects of the workplace on employee health.

The Food and Drug Administration (FDA), another DHHS agency, is mandated to protect consumer health from tainted foods and hazardous drugs, but also conducts research into the effects of radiation upon worker health through its Bureau of Radiological Health. Because the bureau is responsible for regulating emissions from appliances and medical equipment, it studies the biological effects of ionizing and nonionizing radiation.

Research into health hazards in the environment and the setting of standards for limiting such hazards occupies the attention of several federal agencies that are not tied to the DHHS. The most important of these is the EPA, which bears responsibility for promulgating standards and regulations to protect public health and preserve the nation's environment. As its primary task, it regulates the emission of hazardous materials into the atmosphere and discharges into water.

Other departments and agencies conduct research in this area. The Department of Energy (DOE) has undertaken research on the development of cleaner and safer energy. The Department of Agriculture has studied the effects of pesticides and germicides on humans. Through the National Bureau of Standards, the Department of Commerce has developed advanced measuring techniques to monitor environmental pollutants. In the Department of Interior, the Fish and Wildlife service and the Office of Research and Technology have supported a wide range of environmental research. The Department of Defense has tried to identify health hazards emanating from its own facilities and activities. The National Science Foundation has funded research to identify, measure, and assess the impact of hazardous chemicals on the environment and human health. The Nuclear Regulatory Commission has given some attention to the possible hazards of radioactive sources and other problems relating to the operation of nuclear power plants. The National Aeronautics and Space Administration has investigated the harmful effects of noise. The Department of Transportation has supported research to control vehicle noise and emissions. Finally, the Veterans' Administration has done research on the effects of radiation and noise upon the health of humans; in particular, it has undertaken study of the effects of environmental agents upon the pulmonary system.

The research conducted by these agencies is not specifically addressed to problems encountered in the workplace. However, findings in one area often have bearing on others. To assist in the transfer of information and to encourage

Table 13: Federal Agency Support for Environmental Health Research and Related Programs

	Funding (in $ millions) For		
	1977	1978	1979
Department of Health and Human Services	284.3	328.6	339.3
Department of Energy	115.7	126.0	123.7
Environmental Protection Agency	56.2	52.2	69.5
Department of Agriculture	9.9	11.1	11.4
Department of Commerce	10.3	12.7	11.3
Department of Interior	6.7	9.3	10.6
Department of Defense	10.2	6.9	8.6
National Science Foundation	4.7	3.1	5.0
Nuclear Regulatory Commission	1.9	1.8	2.0
National Aeronautics and Space Administration	1.6	1.5	1.6
Department of Housing and Urban Development	0.5	1.6	0.8
Department of Transportation	0.3	0.4	0.3
Veterans Administration	0.3	0.3	0.3
Total	502.6	555.5	584.4

cooperation among agencies, several interagency committees have been formed. These include: the DHHS Committee to coordinate toxicology and related programs; the interagency regulatory liaison group; the EPA/DOE/HHS interagency coordinating committee for energy-related health and environmental effects research; the interagency collaborative group on environmental carcinogenesis; the task force on environmental cancer, heart, and lung diseases; the federal noise effects research panel; and the interagency panel on environmental mutagenesis. Finally, within the Executive Office of the President, the Council on Environmental Quality, the Office of Management and Budget, and the Office of Science and Technology also serve to coordinate the work performed by the various groups.

We now turn to those agencies which play a major role in investigating the effects and in regulating the presence of hazardous substances in the workplace.

The National Institute for Occupational Safety and Health

NIOSH was created in 1970 with the objective of assuring safe and disease-free working conditions for the United States workforce. NIOSH was also granted general research authority under the Public Health Service Act.

Table 14: National Institute for Occupational Safety and Health: Obligations by Object Class (Fiscal Year 1978)

	Direct Operations	Research and Training Grants	Regional Offices	Reimbursements	Total (Including Reimbursements)
Personnel compensation and benefits	16,413,031	—	753,529	2,486,385	19,652,945
Travel and transportation of personnel	1,352,625	—	89,785	270,437	1,712,847
Transportation of things	262,869	—	1,985	7,056	271,910
Rent, communications, and utilities	1,054,233	—	19,477	75,523	1,149,233
Printing and reproduction	948,972	—	2,673	49,467	1,001,112
Other services—total	20,208,782	—	12,582	6,866,877	27,088,241
Supplies and materials	1,468,684	—	9,673	96,790	1,575,147
Equipment	2,712,819	—	5,588	353,745	3,072,152
Lands and structures	15,338	—	—	—	15,338
Grants—total	—	10,900,000	—	—	10,900,000
Insurance claims and indemnities	154	—	—	—	154
Total	44,437,507	10,900,000	895,292	10,206,280	66,439,079

SOURCE: NIOSH.

Table 15: National Institute for Occupational Safety and Health: Direct and Reimbursable Obligations by Selected Program (Dollars in thousands)

Division	Cancer	Criterial Documentation	Mining	Energy
Division of Criteria Documentation and Standards Development		6,420.4		
Division of Respiratory Disease Studies	553.0		335.8	
Division of Surveillance, Hazards Evaluation and Field Studies	4,863.3	73.0		104.5
Division of Biomedical and Behavioral Sciences	2,345.2	331.1		
Division of Physical Science and Engineering	1,580.6	1,081.7		
Division of Technical Services				
Total	9,342.1	7,906.2	335.8	104.5

SOURCE: NIOSH, 1978.

NIOSH conducts research, experiments, and demonstrations to develop criteria that form the basis for recommendations of health and safety standards to the Department of Labor's OSHA. Members of NIOSH were authorized to enter workplaces and examine workers' records and other pertinent documents. The agency also publishes annually a registry of toxic chemicals and their effects. In addition, NIOSH has responsibilities provided for in the Toxic Substance Control Act.

Under the Federal Mine Safety and Health Amendments Act of 1977, NIOSH has further been given authority to conduct research on health problems, recommend standards, and investigate health problems of miners in metal and nonmetal mines, including those who worked in mills and quarries.

Between 1972 and 1974, NIOSH conducted the national occupational hazard survey to determine the extent of worker exposure to chemical substances and physical agents; in all, 4636 workplaces in urban industrial settings were visited. The agency also has undertaken special studies within industries and/or geographical locations to assess workplace conditions.

In 1978 NIOSH had a budget of $66.44 million (see Table 14). The agency spent about $17 million for contract research and services, while another $3.9

Table 15: continued

Respiratory Disease	Women in the Workplace	Technical Services	Behavioral	Total
				6,420.4
3,330.5		1,106.8		5,326.1
	223.3	1,758.6		7,022.7
	742.0		727.8	4,146.1
379.4		759.1		3,800.8
		4,323.5		4,323.5
3,709.9	965.3	7,948.0	727.8	31,039.6

million was for research grants and $7.0 million for manpower development grants.

Its operations may be divided into four major areas: criteria documentation and standards development, research, technical assistance, and manpower development. Under the first category, NIOSH recommends health and safety standards to the Secretary of Labor for promulgation and enforcement. During the 1970s, the agency produced an average of 24 standards annually. As a preliminary step the agency prepares criteria documents, which allow for the determination of the potential or actual harm of industrial processes and classes of substances or, in some cases, individual substances; these documents are then reviewed and transmitted to the Secretary of Labor. In 1978 $7.9 million were devoted to criteria documentation and other standards development.

The second category, applied occupational health and safety research, absorbs the most monies and involves the largest number of employees of any of NIOSH's undertakings. In the main, research is directed at the development or modification of recommended criteria for health and safety standards. The research program itself is organized into seven different categories: occupational carcinogenesis, respiratory disease, reproductive standards, control technology, safety, behavioral aspects, and energy. Funding in areas that are particularly pertinent to this study are given in Table 15.

Occupational Carcinogenesis Program. This program is a comprehensive effort that includes surveillance, industry-wide studies, assessments of the technology used to control exposure, and laboratory research. In the 1970s NIOSH conducted studies on substances like talc, PCB, and styrene-butadiene in industries producing paints, print, and fertilizer, as well as in printing plants and foundries.

Occupational Respiratory Diseases. At NIOSH, research into respiratory disease is conducted at the agency's Morgantown, West Virginia, facility that has long served programs mandated by the Federal Coal Mine Health and Service Act of 1969.

Occupational Hazards Relating to Reproduction. NIOSH attempts to study the effects of hazards in the workplace on both working pregnant women and the fetuses they are carrying. It also seeks to determine if exposure of male workers to industrial hazards has a detrimental effect on their spouses and offspring.

Behavioral. NIOSH investigates the neurotoxic and psychological effects of industrial substances upon workers at risk, and the effects of job stress. Stress is often manifested as cardiovascular and other organic disease.

Energy. Among the energy-producing industries NIOSH focuses upon the non-nuclear ones, although it has given some attention to health and safety hazards in the mining and milling of uranium.

In its capacity as a source of technical assistance, its third major function, NIOSH offers a variety of technical services to employers, employees, universities, and professionals in the field of occupational safety and health. It helps develop model occupational health and safety programs and organizes methods of evaluating hazards. Under this program NIOSH also coordinates the x-ray testing programs mandated by the Coal Act and provides analyses for x-rays taken in the coal mining industry. The agency also operates a clearing house of information. Altogether, technical services absorbed about $9.3 million in 1978. As one of its major functions NIOSH, at the request of employees or employers, conducts health hazard evaluations of workplaces.

Manpower development represents the fourth major category among NIOSH's tasks. About $9.0 million was spent in 1978 for manpower development; the majority of these funds were awarded by grant.

The National Institute of Environmental Health Science

The NIEHS, established in 1966, supports and conducts basic research on the interaction of man and potentially toxic and harmful agents in the environment. In its research the institute emphasizes the need to identify environmental agents and understand the ways in which they act upon biological systems. The institute also conducts epidemiological and toxicological studies.

In 1978 the Office of the Scientific Director was created in NIEHS to oversee and guide the various components of the institute's intramural research program, that is, research organized within the institute proper. The program is composed of several laboratories, including the laboratory of environmental biophysics, the laboratory of environmental toxicology, the laboratory of pharmacology, and the laboratory of environmental mutagenesis, as well as a biometry branch.

The biometry branch conducts applied research in biomathematics, epidemiology, and risk assessment. Its epidemiology program seeks to identify potentially hazardous agents in the environment. The laboratory of environmental biophysics is primarily concerned with the biological effects of physical factors in the environment like nonionizing radiation (microwaves) and noise. At the environmental mutagenesis laboratory researchers evaluate and define the risks to both human somatic and germinal tissue from exposure to genetically active environmental agents. In collaborative research under an interagency agreement, the institute also supports studies to determine the mutagenicity of airborne chemical pollutants and other gases used by industry. Meanwhile, through its research into how toxic substances trigger toxic effects, the laboratory of environmental toxicology is working toward the prevention of environmentally induced diseases. The laboratory tries to identify and understand the ways in which teratogens act, and information about teratogens is stored at the environmental teratology information center.

The NIEHS also supports considerable activity outside its offices through grants, contracts, and training awards (see Table 16) in four areas of primary research: etiology of environmental diseases and disorders, environmental pharmacology and toxicology, environmental pathogenesis and environmental mutagenesis, and reproductive toxicology.

Research sponsored by NIEHS has borne significant results. The institute achieved a major breakthrough with the research it encouraged on the metabolism and pharmacokinetics of chlorinated hydrocarbon chemicals. These studies proved decisive in attaining some control over highly toxic industrial chemicals like the PCBs, and dangerous impurities, including dioxins and furans, that occur in herbicides, disinfectants, soaps, and wood preservatives.

The institute has also served as a resource for regulatory agencies by providing them with information about a host of toxic substances that have been used extensively in the workplace and have at times entered the general environment as well. These include: PBB and PCB; pentachlorophenol and dioxin; asbestos; bis(chloromethyl)ether; diethylstilbestrol; chemical components of air pollution, such as nitrogen dioxide, sulfur dioxide, and carbon monoxide; benzene; methylmercury; and herbicides like 2, 4-D and 2, 4, 5-T.

The scope of NIEHS's work transcends the identification and study of workplace hazards; rather, it extends into all aspects of environmental pollution. However, in many of the institute's programs, research has been conducted into the environmental agents most commonly found in the workplace.

The prediction, detection, and assessment of environmentally caused diseases and disorders program within NIEHS supports research into the nature, location, and extent of environmental pollutants; their relationship to the environment and each other; and the population exposed as a result. Information gained about the behavior of environmental agents in one biological system may make it possible to predict their behavior in other systems. The program has run epidemiological studies of particulate and gaseous pollutants and examined the relationship between acute and chronic lung diseases and such agents as sulfur dioxide, nitrogen dioxide, hydrocarbons, bis(chloromethyl)ether, fluorocarbon polymers, and fiberglass and asbestos. The last four of these agents are used widely in the workplace.

Recently, researchers have turned to the effects of ionizing and nonionizing radiation on the health of those exposed. Funds have been allocated for epidemiological studies of populations that are subjected to radiation and other environmental health hazards at the same time; researchers suspect that the combination may induce a mutagenic or carcinogenic response. New sources of energy also pose new problems. The program may have to set up epidemiological studies to gauge the effects of high voltage electrical transmission, nuclear reactors, disposal of nuclear and toxic waste products, exposure to mine tailings, and radiation from microwaves, radiofrequencies, and ultraviolet light.

The importance of epidemiological studies—retrospective and prospective—has been brought home by findings of asbestosis and lung cancer in shipyard workers, brake repairmen, and others working with materials containing asbestos. The institute has emphasized research by its own investigators into the identification and evaluation of suspected environmental airborne hazards.

Another program within the institute, the mechanisms of environmental diseases and disorders program, promotes research into the means by which harmful agents induce disease. In particular, emphasis has been placed on investigating changes induced by these environmental agents in living organisms and to those that occur in their cells or even the molecules that comprise them. Studies have been made of the effects of environmental agents upon animals and cultures of their organs and tissues; in this way researchers hoped to distinguish the effect of individual agents from those produced by combinations of agents, where synergistic transformations are possible. The actions of mutagenic and carcinogenic substances, among them nitrosamines, aflatoxins, and benzo(a)pyrene, have also been the subject of recent, intensive investigation. Resort to the use of microorganisms, insects, and cultures of cells has improved the speed and sensitivity of the method of assay, or testing, of the mutagenic and carcinogenic potential of these substances, while at the same time reducing the cost.

A further new focus for research conducted by the program has been an evaluation of the effects of a number of environmental agents on male and female reproductive functions and development. These studies have sought to identify sensitive and specific biochemical indicators for developmental and reproductive toxicity.

Among physical factors under investigation, the effects of noise on the cardiovascular function in primates is a major concern. By isolating nerve cells, researchers also hope to evaluate the effects of microwave radiation on the transmission of impulses along neurons.

In addition, research into the effects of radiation has been undertaken to determine whether and by what mechanism radiation might interact with other environmental agents to produce further damaging effects. These studies will supplement a strong research effort aimed at the prediction, detection, and assessment of environmentally induced diseases and disorders in which radiation plays a major part.

Studies of various cellular and tissue alterations produced by environmental carcinogens in pulmonary airways and the co-carcinogenic effects of asbestos and nickel subsulfide are underway, both from a histochemical and ultrastructural perspective.

Finally, the NIEHS allocates about $9 million a year to support nine environmental health science centers, which conduct multidisciplinary research on environmental health problems. Each of these centers has a specific area of investigation assigned to it. Among the designated concerns of these individual centers are: air, water, and food pollution; occupational and industrial neighborhood health and safety; heavy metal toxicity; agricultural chemical hazards; the relationship of the environment to cancer, birth defects, behavioral anomalies, respiratory and cardiovascular diseases, and diseases of other specific organs; and basic aspects of toxicity mechanisms, body defense mechanisms, and the influence of age, nutrition, and other factors in chemically induced injury and disease. Overall, they serve as a national resource for research and manpower development in environmental health science.

The goal of environmental health research is the prevention of disease; to that end, the centers will continue to engage in basic research and develop new data on the metabolism of toxic substances by humans and the means by which molecular and cellular damage occurs. The study of the damage wrought by chemical and mineral agents now in use, or proposed for use, will place emphasis on chemical epidemiology and on a methodology for detecting early symptoms and signs of disease and injury.

The centers have not only made substantive contributions to preventive medicine, but their efforts have also served to clarify the scope of environmental health problems and future needs in this field. Moreover, they have maintained

Table 16: National Institute of Environmental Health Sciences—1979 and 1980 Budget by Program Mechanism

	\multicolumn{6}{c}{Mechanism (Dollars in thousands)}
	\multicolumn{6}{c}{Research Grants}
	Research Projects		Research Centers		Other Research	
Program	1979	1980	1979	1980	1979	1980
Prediction, detection and assessment of environmentally caused diseases and disorders	16,039	13,910	—	—	416	581
Mechanisms of environmental diseases and disorders	12,332	10,912	—	—	184	283
Environmental health research and manpower development resources	—	—	9,567	10,197	—	—
Intramural research	—	—	—	—	—	—
Direct operations and program management	—	—	—	—	—	—
Total obligation	28,371	24,822	9,567	10,197	600	864

SOURCE: NIEHS.

Table 16: continued

Training Programs		Research and Development Contracts		Intramural Research		Direct Operations and Program Management		
Individual and Institutionals								
1979	1980	1979	1980	1979	1980	1979	1980	Total
—	—	5,152	5,152	—	—	—	—	41,250
—	—	3,140	3,140	—	—	—	—	29,991
4,568	6,568	—	—	—	—	—	—	30,900
—	—	—	—	22,223	23,490	—	—	45,713
—	—	—	—	—	—	4,639	4,779	9,418
4,568	6,568	8,292	8,292	22,223	23,490	4,639	4,779	157,272

Mechanism (Dollars in thousands)

efforts to keep pace with changes in industry and technology that may affect environmental health in any number of ways.

The NIEHS publishes a journal entitled: *Environmental Health Perspectives.*

National Cancer Institute

Cancer screening, diagnosis, prevention, and therapy all come within the purview of the NCI. One of its branches, environmental epidemiology, was created in 1975 with the expressed objective of generating and testing ideas about the environmental and host determinants of cancer. This branch was empowered to conduct a broad range of epidemiological studies, in which researchers were to make use of new developments in clinical medicine and oncology, statistical methodology, and carcinogenesis.

Within the branch, the occupational studies section has funded several projects that were undertaken to explain "hot spots," that is, high-risk zones, uncovered by county-by-county surveys of cancer mortality. Moreover, this section has identified subgroups within broad industrial categories who may face high risk of cancer from exposure to carcinogens, and assisted outside agencies or institutions in evaluating the health histories of their workers. In addition, the section has pursued clues of links between cancer and exposure to substances in the workplace provided by animal bioassays and the suggestions of clinicians. The section has also estimated risks associated with known carcinogens in user rather than producer industries. Finally, the section has promoted a variety of methods to obtain information, including use of retrospective cohort and proportionate mortality studies, and data resources from industrial firms, labor unions, professional associations, state vital record departments, the Social Security Administration, and other government agencies.

The National Heart, Lung, and Blood Institute

The Division of Lung Diseases of the NHLBI sponsors some research into occupational respiratory disease. For example, in its fibrotic and immunologic pulmonary diseases program, investigators are studying such respiratory disorders as pigeon breeders disease (hypersensitivity pneumonitis), pulmonary fibrosis, and occupationally induced asthma. Researchers have concentrated their efforts on studying the interaction of the pathogen with the lung and the ways in which the disease takes shape. Basic research has been conducted on animal models, but some clinical studies have made use of specific human populations.

Federal Regulation

The federal agency to which the regulation of the health of workers on the job has been vouchsafed is OSHA. OSHA has moved from being a regulatory agency primarily concerned with problems of safety to one equally concerned with the health of the industrial worker. With most safety regulations already in place, OSHA has shifted its focus to the promulgation of standards and regulations affecting employee health. Through the late 1970s, rules regarding proper record keeping and employee education comprised the better part of OSHA's health regulations. While OSHA has instituted regulations regarding health screening, these tend to be general in nature and minimal in coverage. In the future, however, as new and mounting information about industrial hazards comes to its attention, OSHA is expected to play an increasingly important role in designing a medical screening format for most industrial firms.

Other federal agencies mandated to protect the public against environmental hazards include the EPA, the Nuclear Regulatory Commission, and the Bureau of Radiological Health of the FDA. The EPA, an independent agency, is the watch dog of environmental quality; it often provides information and suggestions to other agencies and the public about occupational health. In fact, trends within the EPA often serve as benchmarks regarding developments within OSHA.

Many businesses have objected to the regulations laid down by OSHA. They have worked through their trade associations to contest standards they find difficult to implement or too costly, or both. Among the trade associations that have played major roles in battling with OSHA are the American Petroleum Institute, the Textile Manufacturers Association, and the Chemical Manufacturers Association.

OSHA's mandate, though, was carefully mapped out in the enabling legislation that established the agency. Under the provisions of the Williams-Steiger Act of 1970 OSHA was created within the Department of Labor to encourage employers and employees to reduce hazards in the workplace and to implement new or improve existing safety and health programs. The act established "separate but dependent responsibilities and rights" for employers and employees in order to achieve better safety and health conditions. It was designed to assure tht job-related injuries and illnesses were accurately and fully reported; to that end, it called for establishing procedures for reporting and record keeping. OSHA was also obliged to develop mandatory job safety and health standards and to enforce them effectively. Until federal standards were fully in place, states were encouraged to establish and administer their own occupational safety and health programs. These programs were meant to be "at least as effective as" the parts of the federal program already in existence.

In line with its mandated responsibilities, OSHA required that all employers of eight employees or more maintain records of occupational injuries and illnesses as they occur. All occupationally induced injuries and illnesses must be recorded if they result in: death (without regard to the length of time between the sustaining of the injury and death or to the length of the illness), one or more lost workdays, restriction of work or motion, loss of consciousness, transfer to another job, or medical treatment beyond first aid. If an on-the-job accident occurs that results in the death of an employee or in the hospitalization of five or more employees, the employer is required to report the details of the accident to the nearest OSHA office within 48 hours.

While record keeping may have increased the cost of doing business for small companies, it has served to bring to light the pernicious effects of previously unidentified substances that cause illness after exposures over long periods of time.

OSHA has been empowered to inspect every establishment covered by the act at any time without advance notice. Alerting an employer in advance of an impending OSHA visit is at least technically punishable by law. Refusal to admit an OSHA compliance officer is similarly punishable.

All rules and regulations formulated or promulgated by OSHA are published in the Federal Register. The agency also publishes a monthly magazine entitled *Job Safety and Health* and various other pamphlets and fact sheets. The agency maintains ten regional offices listed in Appendix A.

The 1970 act establishing OSHA represented a landmark in federal legislation on occupational safety and health. Since then hundreds of issues of environmental safety and health have been brought before Congress, but the strong vested interests of industry, and effective lobbying in their favor, have tended to water down or delay consideration of critical issues. Perhaps the most striking examples of this tendency are the weak or negligible efforts to require the deleading of schools and homes to eliminate the danger of lead poisoning in children, removal of asbestos from public places, and compensation of workers for loss of health and life from exposure at work to hazardous substances. Congress has been mulling over legislation to provide large payments under the worker's compensation program, to revise the product liability laws, and to institute programs for problems arising from exposure to asbestos, lead, and coal dust.

The regulations put forth by OSHA have forced industry to make significant modifications of their operations. As the agency concentrates on issues of health, many more substances and manufacturing processes will be scrutinized. If the legislative picture remains unchanged, industry will face a significant challenge in the 1980s as it begins to try to protect workers' health.

The government has found ways of aiding business in the process. In order to reduce the cost to small and medium-sized companies and to encourage much more substantial compliance with regulations designed to ensure employee safety, the government has instituted several financial aid programs. These include a low-interest loan program administered by the Small Business Administration and available to small companies that can demonstrate "substantial economic injury" in order to comply with OSHA rulings, and a program of plant inspections conducted by OSHA workers without the fear of penalties or charges for noncompliance to assist the small operator in identifying violations.

Education and Training

Occupational medicine is a new—or better—a transformed medical specialty. In the past it commanded low prestige, in part because the duties of the industrial physician were ill-defined and in part because the relationship between workplace and disease was regarded as at best tenuous. The conviction that occupational health and safety hazards endanger the lives of thousands of workers has dramatically changed the role of the industrial physician. The new demand for industrial physicians—and allied health professionals—will be met only if the educational system adjusts to the new reality and establishes educational, training, and certification programs on a national scale.

For its part, NIOSH allocated $8.3 million in 1979 to fund eleven education resource centers throughout the country. The centers provide training programs in occupational medicine, occupational health nursing, industrial hygiene and safety, and continuing education. NIOSH also provided grants in excess of $500,000 in 1978 to several medical schools to train staff in occupational medicine.

Through programs established outside of its designated domains, NIEHS provides training support for young investigators and established scientists who want to study toxicology. NIEHS also administers the National Research Service awards for individual post-doctoral fellows. This program offers fellowships in environmental toxicology, environmental pathology, environmental mutagenesis, environmental epidemiology, and biostatistics.

The upsurge in demand for individuals trained in occupational medicine suggests that more medical students will choose it as their specialty in the future. Before 1975 the number of medical school programs in occupational medicine numbered less than five. By 1975, however, more than ten medical schools provided such programs.

Finally, the federal government has embarked upon an educational program to alert the public to the dangers of exposure to certain substances in both the workplace and community; it also has attempted to increase public awareness of the multiplication of risk that occurs when the smoking of tobacco, the excessive drinking of alcohol, or the use of narcotics is combined with exposure to other hazardous substances. Educational programs also inform affected populations of the availability of health testing services to identify early warning signs of disease. In the late 1970s one such program was initiated for all workers exposed to asbestos at any time during their lives.

LABOR UNIONS

In general, the influence of individual employees in the field of occupational health has been felt through litigation filed for harm suffered. For example, thousands of suits have been filed by victims of asbestos exposure against the major producers of the substance. More than 1500 cases are pending and their number has been on the increase. Although to date the sums won by the plaintiffs have been modest, the total damages sought by all those who have filed are in the billions of dollars.

Labor unions have traditionally fought for the rights of their membership and have, in recent years, grown increasingly responsive to the health concerns of their members. Many of the large international unions have created industrial health departments to address the health hazards posed at work. Unions have also promoted educational and training programs for health professionals interested in occupational medicine.

On occasion, however, unions have joined with manufacturers to oppose the imposing of stringent standards that might result in plant closures and loss of jobs. Some unions have fought attempts by employers to ban employees from smoking cigarettes at work. While the employer has argued that such habits increase the susceptibility of workers to workplace hazards, unions have challenged the ban as an infringement upon the rights of workers. One union tested Johns Manville, the nation's leading producer of asbestos, in court after the company imposed a smoking ban.

Fear of job discrimination against certain employees with health problems limits close cooperation between employers and unions. In many instances, an employee can be deprived of a well-paying job, seniority status, and certain benefits because of a transfer brought on by considerations of health. Some employers may be flexible by assigning jobs in accordance with the rights and benefits won by workers, but this is not general practice.

INDUSTRY PROGRAMS

After fighting for years to ignore the dangers presented by health and safety problems on the job, industry has recently begun to gear up to meet the challenge. The claim of manufacturers that the health of American workers has never been better must be balanced against their establishing in-house medical departments to monitor the health of their employees. The newly found interest in the health of their employees stems from two sources: strengthened federal regulation of occupational health—and the anticipation of even stricter regulation in the future—and fear of liability. A multimillion dollar damage suit was filed in federal District Court in Virginia in the late 1970s against nine asbestos manufacturers by hundreds of shipyard workers who had been exposed to the substance. In its defense the industry faulted the shipyards for not following safety standards by making use of respirators, and needlessly exposing their employees to asbestos dust.

Moreover, the federal government has begun to pressure industry more strongly to maintain workplaces free from health hazards after the harm suffered by workers from exposure to asbestos, Kepone, and PVC came to national attention. Recently, OSHA proposed penalties of up to $359,000 against General Dynamics for health violations at its Groton, Connecticut, plant. The agency accused the company of willfully exposing its workers to hazardous levels of lead, asbestos, and copper.

To avoid conflicts with OSHA and protect themselves against litigation, companies have begun to research this area in depth. For example, Union Carbide began a joint project with NIOSH to study 40,000 former and current employees of three Union Carbide facilities around South Charleston, West Virginia, to determine the effects of chemical exposure on their health. The plants produce chemicals used in insecticides, urethan foams, and coatings for fiber and paper. Also, Exxon Corporation is constructing an environmental health science facility in Somerset County, New Jersey. The facility will test the effects of exposure to petroleum and petrochemical products and will evaluate the work environment in Exxon facilities.

8
Diagnostic and Screening Programs, Equipment and Techniques

Because the body has a limited number of physiopathological responses, occupationally induced disease may not differ in its *clinical manifestations* from naturally occurring disorders. The impetus of an occupational health screening program is to identify early warnings of impending disease and to prevent catastrophic illness from occurring.

The mandate of the surveillance program is to protect the worker from the specific hazards present in the workplace where he is assigned. Therefore, the testing is not a true multiphasic screening approach but, rather, an organ-targeted surveillance program. For instance, if a substance is suspected of being a lung carcinogen, it is unlikely that the screening regimen would include an EKG or urine cytology. However, in the manufacturing industries, and particularly in chemical plants, the workers are exposed to such a variety of potentially hazardous agents that it is both medically and economically feasible to offer workers a truly multiphasic screening program.

The taking of a medical and occupational history has been the common denominator in every medical surveillance program to date. The complete occupational history is very important because many agents do not cause disease until after latent periods that often exceed 20 years. The patient's medical history also includes a description of personal habits and leisure-time activities. This could alone be the cause of abnormal test results, aside from any occupational exposures.

It must be stressed here that all medical surveillance programs outlined in the standards and criteria documents are screening tools, not diagnostic ones. Once an abnormality is detected, further extensive medical evaluations are necessary to identify the origin and nature of the disorder.

Many screening techniques are ideally suited to the occupational medicine field. A list of such tests is shown in Table 17. As we can see, the common specialized tests are audiometry, vision tests, clinical laboratory tests, x-ray and pulmonary function tests. All of the techniques listed are screening approaches and therefore have low sensitivities but high specificities. Sensitivity refers to the percentage of positive tests in the screened population, while specificity relates to the accuracy of the test.

A description of the basic elements of a screening program is given in chapter 6. Here, a detailed discussion of various diagnostic and screening techniques is presented, together with estimates of their utilization in the industrial setting based on the NIOSH and F&S survey data.

Medical surveillance programs vary based on the goal of the project. Industries in which employees are exposed to OSHA-regulated substances provide medical screening programs as recommended by the regulation or the criteria documents. Industries that have few or no workers exposed to hazardous substances provide medical screening that is more geared to identifying early disease, especially cardiovascular disease, hypertension, and diabetes, that is still theoretically preventable or can be treated satisfactorily through medication, diet, or change in personal habits. These latter screening programs are undertaken by industry voluntarily and are devised to save the company money that would be lost due to absenteeism, poor productivity, and loss of valuable personnel. Finally, in some service sectors, such as hospitals, preplacement and periodic medical surveillance is carried out for the protection of the employee as well as the public.

The creation of a full-time company medical department is a desirable first step. Such a department staffed with full-time and part-time interdisciplinary personnel can provide the following services:

full medical support for the management of acute and chronic illness,
first aid and emergency service,
screening regimen for all employees,
rehabilitation services for heart patients or patients with back injuries,
consultation and treatment of alcoholism and mental disease, and
health education.

A company with a large number of employees but many small installations often establishes a full-time medical department at its central facility and provides mobile screening units at the plants located within a reasonable distance. For small plants located far from the central facility, an outside company or a group of physicians are hired to provide the necessary medical services.

The NIOSH study reflecting the 1972-1974 status of health screening in industry reported that only 4 percent of all plants have a formally established medical department. However, such programs covered 31.5 percent of all employees. Moreover, 70 percent of all establishments with 500 employees or more had a formally established medical department (see Table 18). This last result is in agreement with the findings of the F&S survey in that 77 percent of similar sized companies had in-house medical departments (see Table 17). These plants covered 79.6 percent of all employees. So it is evident that the large plants are voluntarily enhancing their ability to serve the needs of their personnel. Where the results are not as encouraging is with the smaller companies. However, it is developments within the smaller companies that will contribute to the growth in the health screening industry.

Testing frequency varied significantly from respondent to respondent. However, the results of the F&S survey, as shown in Table 17, indicate that a large number of plants offer preplacement examinations (55.6 percent) and also a considerable number offer annual examinations (35 percent) to their general employees. Employees in hazardous jobs were given annual examinations by

Table 17: Medical Surveillance Regimens as Reported by All Survey Respondents*

Testing Frequency	General Employees	Employees in Hazardous Jobs
Preemployment only	41.8	13.4
Preemployment and annual	13.8	10.7
Annual	21.2	39.5
Other	22.6	18.3

Type of Tests	% of Respondents
Medical history	92.8
Physical examination	84.8
X-ray	69.5
Pulmonary function	38.9
Clinical laboratory	78.8
Blood	64.8
Urine	78.0
Sputum cytology	10.3
Lead	2.3
Pap smear	2.7
Stool	2.7
EKG	27.5
Audiometry	40.3
Vision tests	31.9
Proctosigmoidoscopy	2.5

*Of those reporting, 77% have a full-time medical department, 11.3% not, and 11.7% did not answer.

SOURCE: F&S Survey.

Table 18: Summary of Number and Percent of Plants and Employees in Plants Covered by Special Medical Services—All Industries

	All Industries				Employees (thousands)			
	Small (8-99)	Medium (100-500)	Large (Over 500)	Total	Small (8-99)	Medium (100-500)	Large (Over 500)	Total
Formally established health unit	15,390 (2.3)	8,163 (13.6)	6,030 (70)	29,583 (4.0)	511.9 (3.3)	1,988.8 (18.4)	9,539.1 (79.6)	12,049.8 (31.5)
Regularly record health information about new employees	341,211 (50.9)	47,653 (79.6)	8,298 (96.3)	397,161 (53.7)	9,322.3 (60.6)	8,926.4 (82)	11,734.9 (97.7)	29,983.7 (78.4)
Require preplacement physical examinations	100,502 (15)	26,513 (44.3)	6,467 (75.0)	133,482 (18.1)	2,954.2 (19.2)	5,324.6 (48.9)	9,986.8 (83.3)	18,265.6 (47.7)
Provide periodic medical examinations	59,546 (8.9)	15,664 (26.2)	4,734 (54.9)	79,944 (10.8)	1,876.2 (12.2)	3,184.6 (29.3)	7,838.6 (65.4)	12,899.5 (33.7)
Provide audiometric examinations	26,008 (3.9)	7,553 (12.6)	2,666 (30.9)	36,227 (4.9)	803.4 (5.2)	1,500.8 (13.8)	5,763.6 (48.1)	8,067.8 (21.1)
Provide periodic pulmonary function screening	15,501 (2.3)	4,438 (7.4)	1,513 (17.6)	21,452 (2.9)	529.3 (3.4)	919.6 (8.4)	3,725 (31.1)	5,174 (13.5)
Provide ophthalmological examinations	32,283 (4.8)	8,232 (13.8)	2,903 (33.7)	43,419 (5.9)	1,027.8 (6.7)	1,719.6 (15.8)	5,774 (48.2)	8,521.4 (22.3)
Provide x-ray examinations	42,428 (6.3)	10,913 (18.2)	3,646 (42.3)	56,988 (7.7)	1,318.3 (8.6)	2,221.8 (20.4)	6,005.3 (50.1)	9,545.4 (24.9)
Provide periodic urine tests	15,076 (2.2)	4,387 (7.3)	1,906 (22.1)	21,369 (2.9)	476.7 (3.1)	918.5 (8.4)	4,109.9 (34.4)	5,505.1 (14.4)
Provide periodic blood tests	19,277 (2.9)	4,062 (6.8)	2,059 (23.9)	25,400 (3.4)	548.6 (3.6)	855.2 (7.9)	4,218.4 (35.2)	5,622.2 (14.7)

Table 19: Performer of Medical Screening and Medical Equipment in Place as Reported by the Survey Respondents

	Percent of 466 Respondents
Current Performer of Tests	
Company medical department	80.6
Single outside provider	21.0
Multiple outside providers	21.6
All of the above	6.4
Future Performer of Tests	
In-house resources	65.2
Outside providers	17.7
Both	7.2
Equipment Available in Situ*	
Audiometer	47.6
Pulmonary function	41.8
EKG	39.5
Stress testing	3.0
Vision tests	38.6
Tonometry	7.3
X-ray	34.1
Clinical laboratory	16.0
Urine	6.2
Blood	4.7
Sigmoidoscope-proctoscope	3.2

*Excludes hospitals.
SOURCE: F&S Survey.

50.2 percent of the plants contributing to the F&S survey. Also 11.1 percent of the plants offered twice-a-year tests for those exposed to hazardous substances.

The NIOSH survey estimated that 18.1 percent of all plants require preplacement examinations and 75 percent of all plants with 500 or more workers require such tests. This survey also estimates that only 10.8 percent of all plants provided periodic examinations and 54.9 percent of all plants with 500 or more workers provided such examinations. This is in line with the F&S findings that indicate that 51.8 percent of such plants provided periodic examinations to general employees.

The majority of the plants (80.6 percent) responding to the F&S survey performed most medical tests in in-house medical departments. However, only 65.2 percent said they intended to do so in the future. Equipment available at

Table 20: Equipment and Techniques in Which New Developments Are Encouraged by the Respondents to the F&S Survey

Type of Equipment	% of Respondents
Computers	7.8
Pulmonary function equipment	6.5
Clinical laboratory technique	5.5
Audiometers	4.1
Chest x-rays	3.7
EKG and stress testing	3.9
Computerized EKG	1.0
Vision tests	2.4
Tonometry	1.2
Physical therapy	1.4
Whirlpool	1.0
A standardized technique to measure strength, stamina and agility	0.08

plant medical departments is listed in Table 19. Equipment that the respondents considered valuable for their practice and either expressed the intention to acquire or hoped to see improved is listed in Table 20.

Other responses in terms of equipment include: unidose packaging, better and cheaper noninvasive multiphasic screening techniques, better portable equipment, microfilm facility, inexpensive defibrillator, breath analyzer, blood pressure measurements, neurological electronic instruments, drug monitoring techniques, and back x-ray system.

Several respondents offered some suggestions other than instrumentation, such as better service, psychiatric consultation, alcohol and drug abuse program, protocols for screening persons exposed to specific hazards, better use of RNs, availability of statistical mortality data and epidemiological studies, breakthroughs in the prediction of chronic disease, and use of paramedics and physician assistants.

LUNG FUNCTION SCREENING AND DIAGNOSIS

With the exception of blood pressure measurements and audiometry, lung function testing is the most common screening procedure in occupational medicine. Table 21 lists the substances that pose hazards requiring pulmonary function screening of exposed workers. NIOSH requires that workmen exposed to certain substances undergo pulmonary function testing. These substances have been starred in Table 21.

Lung function testing is ideally suited for mass screening applications. The procedure is totally noninvasive, relatively easy to perform, and, unlike other screening procedures such as x-ray, poses no health hazard if repeated frequently. Since respiratory disease accounts for approximately half of all cases of serious occupational disease, lung function screening is both necessary and prevalent. For instance, 184 respondents to the F&S survey mentioned lung function testing as part of their screening regimen. This represents 38.7 percent of the total respondents (see Table 17). Moreover 36 respondents from the chemical industry included pulmonary function in their screening regimen. This number represents 64.2 percent of the total chemical establishments responding to the survey.

In addition most respondents, such as corporate physicians, physicians with insurance companies, and others performing executive health tests have included pulmonary evaluations as part of the annual examination. Also, 71.4 percent of all consultants in the occupational medical field who responded to the survey listed pulmonary function as one of the screening tests that they perform on routine examinations of workmen.

The NIOSH survey[42] conducted in the 1972-1974 period estimated that only 4.2 percent of all plants in the manufacturing industries provided pulmonary function to their employees and 3,585,225 or 23.6 percent of all employees underwent such testing.

The F&S survey results, as shown in Table 17, reveal a rather different picture. It must be kept in mind, however, that the respondents to the F&S survey represented mostly facilities employing 500 persons and over. When this fact is taken into account, the results of the NIOSH and F&S surveys are closer (33.7 percent versus 38.9 percent).

Additionally, 6.5 percent of the F&S survey respondents said that they have been reviewing the pulmonary function field with the intention of acquiring devices in this area.

Pulmonary function screening is usually accomplished by the spirometer. Such an instrument measures and calculates the following:

Forced vital capacity (FVC) (measured)
Forced expiratory volume in one second (FEV_1) (measured)
Forced expiratory flow into the midrange ($FEF_{25-75\%}$) (calculated)
Forced end-expiratory flow ($FEF_{75-85\%}$)
Peak expiratory flow rate (PEFR)
Forced expiratory flow between 200-1200 ml ($FEF_{200-1200\ ml}$),
Maximum voluntary ventilation.

Most common tests performed in a screening program of industrial workers are the FVC and FEV_1 tests. FVC is of value in the detection of restrictive pulmonary disease and FEV_1 is used to detect obstructive pulmonary disease.

More sophisticated tests are controversial regarding their value as screening tools. The $FEF_{200-1200}$ reveals the state of the larger airways but it is not as valuable a diagnostic measurement because it is very subjective. On the other hand, the $FEF_{25-75\%}$ provides information on the smaller airways and the $FEF_{75-85\%}$ is valuable in evaluating distal airways.

Other screening tests to assess pulmonary function include: lung volume determinations by nitrogen washout, determinations of lung diffusing capacity, and helium-oxygen spirometry. Although these tests are far more diagnostic in value, they are difficult to perform and are therefore impractical for mass screening applications.

Recently, the radionuclides ^{133}Xe and ^{85}Kr have been used in the early diagnosis of emphysema and black lung disease or whenever airway patency is in question. The patient inhales the radioactive gas mixed with air in a closed system and holds his breath for 35 seconds, by which time all the areas of the lungs are completely ventilated and a scintophotograph is obtained with a gamma camera. The patient breathes normally while other scintophotographs are taken. Then the lungs are cleared of the radionuclide by breathing fresh air and scintograms are taken. Any obstruction in the airways appears at this time as a hot spot on the scintogram. All radioactivity should clear from the lungs in five minutes.

In the past five years significant strides have been made by equipment manufacturers to produce rugged and reliable spirometers to be used in mass screening applications. In 1978 the American Thoracic Society adopted recommendations for spirometric equipment in cooperation with NIOSH. These recommendations served to identify a few acceptable devices among a sea of products that at one time numbered some 55 models.

There are numerous manufacturers of pulmonary function testing equipment. Several of those that have advertised their products or participated in trade shows specifically addressed to the occupational medicine field are listed in chapter 10. Several respondents to the F&S survey included the trade name of the devices they use. Among those mentioned (and the number of respondents) were: Jones Pulmonor (15), Vitalograph (4), Ohio (4), Warren E. Collins (2), Cavitron (1), LSE (3), and SRL (1).

As discussed, devices to assess pulmonary function in occupational medicine are primarily spirometers. There are two types of spirometers, volume or flow measuring devices. Volume measuring spirometers are simple, reliable, and generally less expensive than flow measuring units. However, they have declined somewhat in popularity due to the fact that they are generally cumbersome to move around and often do not incorporate automated techniques to obtain desired calculations. Bellows type spirometers are the simplest to use and the least expensive, with prices ranging from $260 to $900. These devices provide a permanent chart recording of the test results. Spirometers in this category include the Breon, Vitalor (Air Shields, Inc.), and Vitalograph units. A more expensive

Table 21: Exposure Hazards that Require Lung Function Tests

Acrylamide	Fibrous glass
Acrylonitrile	Fluorides, inorganic
*Allyl chloride	Fluorocarbon decomposition products
Alkanes	Formaldehyde
Ammonia	Hot environments
Arsenic	Hydrogen fluoride
Asbestos	Hydrogen sulfide
Asphalt fumes	Isopropyl alcohol
Benzoyl peroxide	Malathion
*Benzyl chloride	Methyl chloride
*Beryllium	Methyl parathion
*Boron trifluoride	*Nickel, inorganic and compounds
*Cadmium	*Nickel carbonyl
Carbaryl	*Nitriles
*Carbon black	Nitric acid
Carbon dioxide	*Nitrogen oxides
Carbon monoxide	Ozone
Chromic acid	Phenol
Chlorine	*Phosgene
Chloroform	Refined petroleum solvent
*Chloroprene	*Silica, crystalline
Chromium (VI)	Sodium hydroxide
*Coal tar products (coal tar, creosote, coal tar pitch)	Sulfuric acid
Coke oven emissions	*Sulfur dioxide
Compressed air atmospheres	Tetrachloroethylene
*Cotton dust	*Toluene and other diisocyanates
Cyanide (hydrogen, cyanide salts)	1, 1, 1, -Trichloroethane
DBCP	Trichloroethylene
Dinitro-ortho-cresol	*Tungsten and cemented tungsten carbide
Dioxane	*Vanadium
Epichlorohydrin	Xylene
Ethylene dibromide	Zinc oxide
Ethylene dichloride	

*Required by OSHA.

Table 22: Number and Percent of Plants and Employees in Plants Covered by Periodic Pulmonary Function Tests for Employees

Code	Industry	Small (8-99)	Medium (100-500)	Large (Over 500)	Total
20	Food and kindred products	285 (2.2)	379 (12.7)	95 (23.5)	759 (4.7)
21	Tobacco products	—	—	15 (37.5)	15 (7.7)
22	Textile mill products	108 (4.0)	—	8 (21.6)	115 (3.6)
23	Apparel and other textile products	249 (1.9)	—	—	249 (1.6)
24	Lumber and wood products	112 (4.0)	—	13 (37.1)	125 (4.0)
25	Furniture and fixtures	26 (0.7)	18 (2.6)	10 (13.2)	55 (1.2)
26	Paper and allied products	30 (0.9)	30 (2.1)	25 (12.1)	84 (1.7)
27	Printing and publishing	67 (0.6)	—	—	67 (0.5)
28	Chemicals and allied products	600 (11.2)	64 (6.9)	118 (25.3)	781 (11.6)
29	Petroleum and coal products	27 (3.9)	56 (23.8)	56 (88.9)	140 (14.1)
30	Rubber and miscellaneous plastics	358 (7.9)	70 (7.1)	24 (16.2)	452 (8.0)
31	Leather and leather products	—	—	—	—
32	Stone, clay and glass products	635 (10.0)	190 (13.2)	31 (21.7)	856 (10.8)
33	Primary metals	105 (2.8)	92 (10.0)	138 (38.0)	335 (6.6)
34	Fabricated metals	819 (4.9)	175 (6.6)	10 (2.5)	1,000 (5.1)
35	Machinery, except electrical	35 (0.3)	77 (4.1)	155 (26.8)	267 (1.9)
36	Electric and electronic equipment	43 (1.4)	59 (3.9)	146 (31.5)	248 (4.9)
37	Transportation equipment	32 (1.3)	35 (5.7)	98 (26.4)	166 (4.8)
38	Instruments	14 (0.4)	14 (3.8)	2 (1.0)	30 (0.8)
39	Miscellaneous manufacturing	45 (0.9)	21 (2.9)	50 (52.6)	116 (2.0)

Table 22: continued

Code	Industry	Small (8–99)	Medium (100–500)	Large (Over 500)	Total
20	Food and kindred products	20 (5.4)	102 (14.7)	109 (32.5)	231 (16.5)
21	Tobacco products	—	—	21 (32.1)	21 (26.1)
22	Textile mill products	2 (2.0)	—	7 (15.6)	8 (3.7)
23	Apparel and other textile products	13 (2.5)	—	—	13 (1.4)
24	Lumber and wood products	2 (2.1)	—	12 (44.7)	14 (8.5)
25	Furniture and fixtures	2 (1.5)	3 (2.2)	9 (16.8)	14 (4.6)
26	Paper and allied products	1 (1.2)	4 (1.5)	41 (23.0)	47 (8.2)
27	Printing and publishing	6 (1.7)	—	—	6 (0.5)
28	Chemicals and allied products	25 (12.6)	20 (10.2)	292 (50.5)	337 (34.9)
29	Petroleum and coal products	1 (5.1)	15 (27.8)	118 (96.8)	134 (68.5)
30	Rubber and miscellaneous plastics	3 (2.0)	20 (10.5)	89 (43.6)	112 (21.0)
31	Leather and leather products	—	—	—	—
32	Stone, clay and glass products	21 (11.8)	53 (17.2)	124 (58.2)	198 (28.3)
33	Primary metals	5 (4.4)	25 (11.2)	708 (70.5)	738 (54.8)
34	Fabricated metals	31 (7.0)	43 (8.3)	7 (1.8)	81 (6.0)
35	Machinery, except electrical	2 (0.9)	16 (4.2)	312 (34.7)	330 (21.5)
36	Electric and electronic equipment	3 (2.7)	15 (4.6)	756 (70.6)	774 (51.6)
37	Transportation equipment	0.5 (0.7)	6 (3.9)	451 (45.1)	458 (37.4)
38	Instruments	1 (1.5)	1 (2.1)	6 (2.5)	8 (2.2)
39	Miscellaneous manufacturing	1 (0.9)	6 (4.0)	53 (56.9)	60 (15.8)

SOURCE: NIOSH Occupational Hazards Survey, 1977.

bellows unit is the Jones Pulmonor II and its companion microprocessor that allows automated recording of several test variables and offers an interpretation of the test subject's condition. The total package can cost upward of $6100.

Another type of volume measuring device is the water-sealed spirometer, which is also simple to operate, accurate, and relatively maintenance free. Devices based on this principle include the Stead-Wells unit (Warren E. Collins) and the Collins Survey Spirometer (Warren E. Collins). Prices for these devices range from $3000 to $3800. Another type of spirometer similar in operation to the water-seal type is the dry rolling seal device, except that it uses a rolling plastic seal instead of water. Such spirometers are marketed by Ohio Medical and Cardio-Pulmonary Instruments, Inc. Prices in this category are estimated from $990 to $4000 for units incorporating microprocessors.

Flow measuring spirometers are more expensive and, unless properly maintained and calibrated, less accurate than the volume measuring devices. However, they are portable, easy to operate, and automated, which makes them uniquely suitable for mass screening applications. Such devices include the Cavitron SC-20 and the Vanguard (LSE). Prices range from $3000 to $6000, depending on features and automation capabilities.

Important features of pulmonary function testing equipment destined for the occupational health screening market are ease of use (minimal maintenance problems) and the capability for the equipment to provide a permanent record of all test variables.

The market outlook for these devices in occupational medicine applications is excellent. They are expected to be an integral part of all periodic screening in the hazardous industries. One group of companies most likely to become a major user of pulmonary function equipment are the manufacturing establishments. Overall, NIOSH estimates that only 4.2 percent of all plants offer pulmonary function testing to their employees and that only 23.6 percent of all employees undergo such tests. Moreover only 21.8 percent of large plants (500 or more employees) offer such tests to 43.5 percent of all the workers employed by such plants. The penetration of this type of testing is best illustrated in Table 22, which lists the various types of manufacturing groups. More detailed analysis of the trends within each group is given in chapter 9.

X-RAYS

X-ray tests are one of the most widely used screening procedures in occupational medicine. Many surveillance standards require chest x-rays, as shown in Table 23.

Chest x-ray examinations are performed to detect various diseases, such as tuberculosis, lung cancer, and asymptomatic chronic lung disease. X-rays for tuberculosis screening are not justified unless performed in a high-risk population (hospital personnel, for instance). Routine chest x-rays are also not cost effective in the early detection of lung cancer. X-rays should be performed on workers exposed to hazardous substances that affect pulmonary function to detect early asymptomatic chronic lung disease.

A preplacement chest x-ray is justified because it allows the physician to document the pulmonary status of the new employee and to recommend appropriate workplace environment; it is, in fact, a base-line record for future reference, and comparison.

Spinal x-rays are recommended during a preemployment physical only if the employer's experience confirms their value. Such x-rays should never be performed on a routine basis.

Currently, there is widespread concern regarding the overutilization of x-rays. Overutilization, for the purposes of this study, will be examined only as it applies to excessive examinations per patient. Other sources of overutilization include excessive exposure to radiation due to equipment or technician errors or excessive number of films taken. Investigations to establish the safety of x-ray procedures, often to be performed twice yearly according to some standards, have not been carried out.

Generally, occupational physicians are encouraged to use x-ray tests sparingly and to develop criteria regarding the frequency of such tests and to define the categories of workers that would benefit from them. Also, physicians are encouraged to use other techniques (pulmonary function, sputum cytology) whenever possible to avoid unnecessary exposure to radiation.

Table 23: Substances in the Workplace Requiring X-Ray Testing of Workers

Acrylonitrile	Hydrazines*
Antimony	4, 4'-Methylene-bis (2-chloroaniline)
Arsenic	Nickel carbonyl
Asbestos	Nitric acid
Benzyl chloride	Nitriles
Beryllium	Organotin compounds
Carbon black	Ozone
Chlorine	Phosgene
Chloroprene	Silica
Chromium	Toluene diisocyanate
Coal tar products (coal tar, creosote, coal tar pitch)	Tungsten and cemented tungsten carbide
Coke oven emissions	Vanadium
Diisocyanates	

*Male pelvic examination.

Table 24: Number and Percent of Plants and Employees in Plants Covered by Periodic Chest X-Rays for Employees

Code	Industry	Small (8–99)	Plants Medium (100–500)	Large (Over 500)	Total
20	Food and kindred products	1,921 (15.0)	1,108 (37.2)	181 (44.8)	3,210 (19.8)
21	Tobacco products	—	86 (17.3)	15 (37.5)	15 (7.7)
22	Textile mill products	134 (5.0)	256 (11.0)	18 (48.6)	237 (7.3)
23	Apparel and other textile products	426 (3.2)	27 (9.7)	—	683 (4.4)
24	Lumber and wood products	141 (5.1)	19 (2.8)	13 (37.1)	181 (5.9)
25	Furniture and fixtures	91 (2.4)	349 (24.8)	10 (13.2)	120 (2.6)
26	Paper and allied products	177 (5.5)	167 (11.2)	48 (23.3)	574 (11.8)
27	Printing and publishing	67 (0.6)	234 (25.4)	112 (30.4)	345 (2.5)
28	Chemicals and allied products	840 (15.7)	107 (45.5)	210 (45.0)	1,284 (19.0)
29	Petroleum and coal products	89 (12.8)	153 (15.6)	56 (88.9)	253 (25.5)
30	Rubber and miscellaneous plastics	1,301 (28.8)	21 (4.8)	65 (43.9)	1,518 (26.9)
31	Leather and leather products	62 (5.3)	424 (29.5)	—	83 (5.0)
32	Stone, clay and glass products	368 (21.5)	219 (23.8)	31 (21.7)	1,824 (22.9)
33	Primary metals	293 (7.8)	360 (13.6)	284 (78.2)	796 (15.8)
34	Fabricated metals	599 (3.6)	374 (20.2)	142 (35.1)	1,101 (5.6)
35	Machinery, except electrical	268 (2.3)	163 (10.8)	247 (42.7)	889 (6.3)
36	Electric and electronic equipment	128 (4.1)	84 (13.6)	214 (46.2)	506 (10.0)
37	Transportation equipment	115 (4.7)	62 (16.9)	134 (36.1)	333 (9.6)
38	Instruments	58 (1.8)	60 (8.3)	34 (17.3)	153 (4.0)
39	Miscellaneous manufacturing	90 (1.8)	60 (8.3)	50 (52.6)	200 (3.5)

Table 24: continued

Code	Industry	Small (8-99)	Employees in Plants (thousands) Medium (100-500)	Large (Over 500)	Total
20	Food and kindred products	84 (22.3)	258 (37.3)	123 (36.8)	465 (33.2)
21	Tobacco products	—	—	21 (32.1)	21 (26.1)
22	Textile mill products	3 (3.2)	26 (27.2)	12 (28.4)	41 (17.9)
23	Apparel and other textile products	20 (4.0)	45 (12.0)	—	65 (7.1)
24	Lumber and wood products	4 (4.9)	5 (9.8)	12 (44.7)	21 (13.0)
25	Furniture and fixtures	5 (4.4)	5 (3.9)	9 (16.8)	19 (6.4)
26	Paper and allied products	8 (6.1)	66 (25.1)	66 (37.1)	141 (24.6)
27	Printing and publishing	6 (1.7)	56 (18.1)	160 (27.7)	223 (18.0)
28	Chemicals and allied products	38 (19.5)	57 (30.0)	352 (60.9)	448 (46.4)
29	Petroleum and coal products	4 (22.4)	27 (49.9)	118 (96.8)	149 (76.3)
30	Rubber and miscellaneous plastics	21 (15.0)	41 (21.5)	132 (64.5)	194 (36.3)
31	Leather and leather products	1 (2.7)	4 (4.5)	—	5 (3.4)
32	Stone, clay and glass products	44 (24.4)	115 (37.7)	124 (58.2)	284 (40.5)
33	Primary metals	9 (7.4)	57 (25.8)	940 (93.6)	1,006 (74.7)
34	Fabricated metals	19 (4.3)	95 (18.3)	137 (35.6)	251 (18.6)
35	Machinery, except electrical	14 (5.0)	74 (20.0)	395 (43.9)	483 (31.4)
36	Electric and electronic equipment	8 (8.3)	38 (11.6)	829 (77.4)	875 (58.3)
37	Transportation equipment	5 (6.3)	20 (13.7)	626 (62.6)	651 (53.2)
38	Instruments	3 (4.0)	12 (17.2)	38 (16.6)	53 (13.9)
39	Miscellaneous manufacturing	2 (1.7)	13 (8.4)	53 (56.9)	68 (17.8)

SOURCE: NIOSH Occupational Hazard Survey, 1977.

Most x-ray testing is performed outside the plant facility, either by a hospital, health maintenance organization, or private laboratory. However, large plants also have simple equipment in situ. Probably the x-ray system is the single most expensive item in a multiphasic screening installation. Therefore we expect that such tests will continue to be performed outside the plant at high volume testing services that can justify the use of x-ray equipment.

The NIOSH survey[42] estimated that 7.7 percent of all industrial facilities offered some type of x-ray screening to their employees. It also estimated that 42.3 percent of plants employing 500 or more offered such tests (see Table 18). X-ray examinations were part of the regimen of 69.5 percent of the respondents to the F&S survey. This indicates a significant increase in the utilization of x-rays, since the NIOSH survey estimated that only 42.3 percent of plants with more than 500 workers provided periodic x-ray examinations. Moreover, 34.1 percent reported having x-ray equipment in situ, and another 3.7 percent have been considering use of such equipment.

X-rays will continue to be one of the primary screening techniques available to the occupational specialist. Certain industries are expected to use such tests more widely than others. Table 24 illustrates the use of x-rays in the manufacturing industry, as estimated by NIOSH.

HEARING TESTS

As expected, audiometry is one of the most common medical testing procedures offered by industry. Since hearing problems represent the largest single occupationally induced disorder, most industries where noise exposure is a factor offer periodic hearing tests to all exposed workers. Audiometric examinations are performed to identify those with hearing problems during preplacement examination, to detect early warnings of problems during periodic examinations, and to assess the effectiveness of the hearing conservation program.

Although audiometry is relatively simple to perform, it must be carried out by experienced personnel, since many factors can interfere and produce unacceptable results. A NIOSH survey conducted in the mid 1970s showed that 80 percent of the companies that performed audiometric tests used inadequate testing equipment.

Screening audiometry is at best an inexact approach to early detection of subtle hearing loss trends. Although a soundproof booth is not absolutely necessary, it helps avoid errors due to surrounding sounds. During an audiometric procedure, a headset is placed over the subjects' ears and 500 Hz tone is introduced at a comfortable hearing level. The patient signals when he hears it. Then the tone is decreased by five decibels at a time until the patient signals that he cannot hear it anymore. Then the process is repeated from the inaudible level until the tone can be heard again by the subject. In this way a descending and an ascending threshold are obtained. This procedure is repeated at 1000, 2000, and 4000 Hz. Then the decibel values at each frequency tested are plotted to ascertain any hearing deficiencies. Noise-induced hearing loss (sensorineural) usually results in diminished hearing capacity at high frequencies.

More sophisticated devices, such as pure-tone audiometers utilized in a soundproof chamber, can provide much more accurate information, evaluating both air and bone conduction in a frequency range of 125-8000 Hz.

Prices for simple screening audiometers start at about $150.00. Sophisticated automated units cost from $1000 to $30,000 for a motorized multistation testing unit.

Nearly 47.6 percent of the respondents to the F&S survey indicated that their plants (or offices) have an audiometer available on the site. Also 40.3 percent of the respondents indicated that they provide periodic audiometric screening. The higher percentage of those owning a device as compared to those providing the screening is attributed to the fact that many service companies that provide screening to industry, and therefore have audiometers in their laboratories, do not screen any of their own employees.

Also, 4.1 percent of the respondents to the F&S survey expressed plans to acquire audiometers in the near future and said they would like to see more reliable and automated devices.

NIOSH estimates (see Table 18) that 4.9 percent of all plants provide periodic examinations and 30.9 percent of plants with more than 500 employees offer such tests.

Audiometers must be designed to meet the American National Standard Specification for Audiometers (ANSI A 3.6-1969). There are numerous manufacturers of audiometers.

Beltone (1 percent) and Maico (0.6 percent) were mentioned by name by the respondents of the F&S survey owning such devices. Other manufacturers of audiometers are listed in chapter 10.

Table 25 shows the NIOSH estimates regarding the use of audiometry in manufacturing plants.

CARDIOVASCULAR SCREENING AND ALLIED PRODUCTS

Cardiovascular screening is a standard test in executive health evaluations and is often performed routinely in patients older than 40 years of age. It mainly consists of an EKG, but some companies have also included stress-testing and Holter monitoring procedures to be employed in selected cases.

Exposure to only a few OSHA-regulated substances (antimony, carbon black) requires an electrocardiogram and although some employers offer EKG screening at preplacement, this examination is not a test performed to protect workers from occupational exposures per se. Actually, it is theorized that work-related

Table 25: Number and Percent of Plants and Employees in Plants Covered by Periodic Audiometric Examinations for Employees

Code	Industry	Small (8–99)	Plants Medium (100–500)	Large (Over 500)	Total
20	Food and kindred products	615 (4.81)	574 (19.3)	160 (39.6)	1,348 (8.3)
21	Tobacco products	—	5 (14.7)	25 (62.5)	30 (15.3)
22	Textile mill products	166 (6.2)	62 (12.5)	8 (21.6)	236 (7.3)
23	Apparel and other textile products	383 (2.9)	—	14 (31.8)	397 (2.6)
24	Lumber and wood products	176 (6.3)	17 (6.1)	13 (37.1)	206 (6.7)
25	Furniture and fixtures	37 (1.0)	57 (8.4)	43 (56.6)	136 (2.9)
26	Paper and allied products	213 (6.6)	379 (26.9)	62 (30.1)	653 (13.4)
27	Printing and publishing	—	78 (5.2)	69 (18.7)	147 (1.1)
28	Chemicals and allied products	516 (9.6)	189 (20.5)	255 (54.6)	959 (14.2)
29	Petroleum and coal products	43 (6.2)	72 (30.6)	56 (88.9)	171 (17.2)
30	Rubber and miscellaneous plastics	1,224 (27.1)	81 (8.3)	14 (9.5)	1,319 (23.4)
31	Leather and leather products	—	—	3 (0.2)	3 (0.2)
32	Stone, clay and glass products	598 (9.4)	214 (14.9)	31 (21.7)	844 (10.6)
33	Primary metals	135 (3.6)	215 (23.3)	263 (72.5)	613 (12.2)
34	Fabricated metals	1,480 (8.9)	429 (16.3)	80 (19.8)	1,990 (10.1)
35	Machinery, except electrical	227 (1.9)	235 (12.7)	299 (51.7)	762 (5.4)
36	Electric and electronic equipment	89 (2.9)	74 (4.9)	182 (39.3)	345 (6.8)
37	Transportation equipment	—	20 (3.2)	168 (45.3)	188 (5.4)
38	Instruments	14 (0.4)	22 (6.0)	54 (27.4)	89 (2.3)
39	Miscellaneous manufacturing	66 (1.3)	—	9 (9.5)	75 (1.3)

Table 25: continued

Code	Industry	Small (8-99)	Medium (100-500)	Large (Over 500)	Total
20	Food and kindred products	30 (7.9)	144 (20.8)	153 (45.6)	327 (23.3)
21	Tobacco products	—	2 (17.8)	55 (83.7)	57 (70.5)
22	Textile mill products	5 (5.1)	15 (15.1)	7 (15.6)	26 (11.2)
23	Apparel and other textile products	20 (3.9)	—	19 (50.0)	39 (4.2)
24	Lumber and wood products	6 (7.4)	3 (5.4)	12 (44.7)	21 (12.9)
25	Furniture and fixtures	1 (0.9)	12 (9.5)	32 (60.4)	46 (15.5)
26	Paper and allied products	13 (10.2)	75 (28.2)	80 (44.9)	168 (29.5)
27	Printing and publishing	—	24 (7.6)	118 (20.4)	141 (11.4)
28	Chemicals and allied products	22 (11.0)	48 (25.4)	379 (65.5)	449 (46.5)
29	Petroleum and coal products	2 (9.4)	21 (39.0)	118 (96.8)	141 (72.0)
30	Rubber and miscellaneous plastics	18 (12.9)	25 (12.9)	83 (40.4)	125 (23.4)
31	Leather and leather products	—	—	6 (25.1)	6 (4.1)
32	Stone, clay and glass products	23 (12.6)	55 (18.0)	124 (58.2)	202 (28.9)
33	Primary metals	7 (6.0)	55 (24.6)	930 (92.6)	992 (73.6)
34	Fabricated metals	57 (12.7)	99 (19.3)	106 (27.6)	263 (19.5)
35	Machinery, except electrical	4 (1.6)	51 (13.8)	664 (73.8)	719 (46.7)
36	Electric and electronic equipment	5 (5.0)	21 (6.3)	809 (75.6)	835 (55.6)
37	Transportation equipment	—	3 (2.0)	731 (73.1)	734 (60.0)
38	Instruments	714 (0.8)	4 (6.1)	33 (14.7)	38 (10.0)
39	Miscellaneous manufacturing	986 (0.7)	—	8 (8.8)	9 (2.4)

SOURCE: NIOSH Occupational Hazards Survey, 1977.

stress is far more detrimental to the cardiovascular system than exposure to any hazardous substance. Therefore EKG screening is often performed only on personnel working in stressful environments (executives, air controllers) or whose jobs carry life or death responsibilities.

Most of the respondents to the F&S survey who included EKGs in their testing regimens (27.5 percent) generally performed them on patients older than 40 years of age and only rarely on those between 35 and 40 years of age. Also, 39.5 percent reported having EKG equipment available on premises and 3 percent reported having stress testing equipment. Another 3.9 percent of the respondents wanted to see better EKG and stress testing equipment become available because of their intention to acquire such devices and 1 percent said that they were intending to buy computerized EKG systems.

Stress testing has recently become a controversial screening technique and many claim that it is rarely cost effective and should not be carried out in asymptomatic individuals. Exercise testing is only valuable in assessing the level of exercise tolerance in individuals who are to undertake an exercise program.

EKG equipment varies in price from $1500 to $18,000 for computer-assisted devices. Stress testing installations also cost from $3500 to $25,000. Holter systems cost from $13,000 to $18,000.

In addition to screening devices, many companies also have cardiac resuscitation equipment, such as oxygen delivery system and defibrillators. However, respondents to our survey (except for two plants) failed to report having any such systems.

There are numerous suppliers of cardiovascular diagnostic devices. Several manufacturers that have aggressive programs in the occupational medicine marketplace are listed in chapter 10.

The NIOSH survey did not include EKG in its testing regimen and therefore comparisons cannot be drawn. Since most EKG testing is performed in executive examinations, nonmanufacturing industries use this test as frequently as manufacturers.

CLINICAL LABORATORY TESTS

Clinical laboratory tests offer a fast, reliable, and relatively inexpensive medical screening tool. Nearly all disorders have some manifestation in body fluids and all industrial occupational medicine programs use clinical laboratory testing in their employee screening programs.

Clinical laboratory tests provide a means of detecting the presence of a substance in the body or its metabolites. Mere presence, however, does not imply intoxication.

In addition to the standard laboratory tests performed in a general screening procedure, there are more specific tests to evaluate exposure and response to a certain substance. It is estimated that there are more than 2000 metabolites that can be presently detected with existing laboratory techniques.

Clinical laboratory tests are recommended in the medical surveillance programs of many diverse workplaces, depending on the agents present, as can be seen in Table 26. The most common laboratory tests are blood and urine analyses. However, other tests, such as cytology and cancer screening evaluations, are also becoming increasingly popular. Some of the most common laboratory tests performed in occupational medicine programs are discussed in this section in some detail.

Most laboratory procedures, with the exception of some simple screening tests, are sent out by industry to be performed by clinical laboratories.

Generally, it is estimated that laboratory testing is a commonly used screening technique in occupational medicine. Approximately 78.8 percent of all contributors to the F&S survey reported the use of such testing procedures. Also 16 percent of the contributors said that they have some type of laboratory equipment in situ. However, the majority of such tests are performed by outside providers.

Blood Tests

Blood tests are a recommended screening procedure in a variety of industries to evaluate worker exposure to many hazardous substances, as listed in Table 26. Four types of blood sample analyses are common in industrial medicine: blood chemistry, hematology, serology, and analyses for traces of industrial substances.

The NIOSH survey[42] estimates that 3.4 percent of all industries employing 14.7 percent of all workers offered blood screening to its employees. Also, 23.9 percent of all plants employing more than 500 workers per plant and representing a total of 35.2 percent of such workers provided periodic blood tests (see Table 18). In the manufacturing industries this study reported that an estimated 5 percent of all plants representing 24.1 percent of all workers provided periodic tests to their employees. Moreover 25.5 percent of all manufacturing plants with 500 or more employees representing 43.1 percent of all workers employed by plants of that size provided such examinations periodically (see Table 28).

The F&S survey produced different results, with 64.8 percent of the companies responding, reporting the availability of periodic blood tests as a part of their medical screening regimen (see Table 17).

Blood chemistries are the most common tests, performed either to screen patients exposed to specific hazards or in general health evaluation procedures (preplacement examinations, executive physicals). Such tests result in qualitative and quantitative information concerning the chemical or metabolic constituents of blood. Blood chemistry tests are performed to monitor workers exposed to OSHA-regulated substances and in multiphasic executive examinations, mostly for the detection of early warnings of heart disease.

Table 26: Substances Requiring Clinical Laboratory Tests

Agent	Type of Test
Acrylonitrile	Fecal occult blood*
Allyl chloride	Blood chemistry Hematology Urinalysis
Arsenic	Blood chemistry
Asbestos	Urinalysis
Benzene	Blood chemistry Hematology
Benzoyl peroxide	Blood chemistry
Beryllium	Blood/urine trace metals Cytology (sputum)
Cadmium	Blood chemistry Urinalysis
Carbaryl	Blood chemistry Urinalysis
Carbon black	Cytology (sputum)
Carbon dioxide	Blood chemistry
Carbon monoxide	Hematology
Chloroform	Blood chemistry Hematology Urinalysis
Chromium	Blood chemistry Blood/urine trace metals Cytology
Coal tar products	Cytology (sputum)
Coke oven emissions	Urinalysis Cytology (sputum)
DBCP	Blood chemistry Urinalysis
Dinitro-ortho-cresol	Blood chemistry Urinalysis
Dioxane	Blood chemistry Urinalysis
Epichlorohydrin	Blood chemistry Hematology Urinalysis

Table 26: continued

Agent	Type of Test
Ethylene dibromide	Blood chemistry Urinalysis
Ethylene dichloride	Blood chemistry
Ethylene oxide	Blood chemistry Urinalysis
Hydrazines	Blood chemistry Urinalysis
Hydrogen fluoride	Blood chemistry Urinalysis Blood/urine trace metals
Hydrogen sulfide	Blood chemistry Cytology
Isopropyl alcohol	Blood chemistry
Kepone	Liver function
Ketones	Urinalysis
Lead	Hematology Urinalysis Blood/urine trace metals
Malathion	Hematology
Mercury	Urinalysis
Methyl parathion	Blood chemistry
4,4'-Methylene-bis	Blood chemistry Urinalysis
Methylene chloride	Hematology Cytology
Nickel carbonyl	Urinalysis
Organotin compounds	Blood chemistry Hematology Urinalysis
Parathion	Blood chemistry Hematology
Pesticides	Blood chemistry Hematology
Phenol	Blood chemistry Urinalysis

(Table 26: continued overleaf)

Table 26: continued

Agent	Type of Test
Polychlorinated biphenyls	Blood chemistry Hematology
Refined petroleum solvent	Blood chemistry Hematology Urinalysis
1, 1, 2, 2-Tetrachloroethane	Blood chemistry Hematology
Tetrachloroethylene	Blood chemistry
Thiols	Blood chemistry Hematology Urinalysis
Toluene	Blood chemistry Hematology
Toluene diisocyanate	Hematology
1, 1, 1-Trichloroethane	Blood chemistry
Trichloroethylene	Blood chemistry Hematology Urinalysis
Vinyl chloride	Blood chemistry Urinalysis
Xylene	Blood chemistry Hematology Urinalysis

*For Special Groups only.

Specialized organ profiles required by OSHA regulations have only been established for liver function evaluations. Since many diverse substances are toxic to the liver, an attempt has been made to devise a screening method, but for all purposes blood chemistry evaluations and other laboratory procedures do not serve as early warnings, since test abnormalities appear only after significant damage has occurred.

Hematology is a recommended screening procedure for workers exposed to numerous OSHA-regulated substances that are suspected of causing disturbances of the hematopoietic system. Blood abnormalities also provide an early warning of occupational disease. Such disorders include many forms of anemia and leukemia. Hematological tests include: total red and white blood cell counts, blood cell differential, hematocrit, hemoglobin, and sedimentation rate.

Table 27: Blood Tests Available to Detect Dangerous Exposures to Workplace Hazards

Tests	Price Range*	Tests	Price Range*
Aluminum	$35.00-$70.00	Iron (serum)	5.00- 45.00
Antimony	18.00- 45.00	Lithium (serum)	6.00- 12.00
Arsenic	15.00- 45.00	Magnesium (serum)	6.50- 22.00
Benzene	115.00	Manganese	18.00- 40.00
Beryllium	21.00- 45.00	Mercury	15.00- 45.00
Bismuth	18.00- 45.00	Molybdenum	35.00- 50.00
Blood lead	5.75- 18.00	Nickel (serum)	25.00- 40.00
Cadmium	10.00- 45.00	Organophosphates	200.00
Calcium	4.50- 6.50	Parathion	
Carbon monoxide	20.00- 25.00	Phenol	25.00- 35.00
Chromium	23.00- 60.00	Potassium	4.00- 5.50
Cobalt	18.00- 30.00	Selenium	21.00- 40.00
Copper	8.00- 22.00	Silver	21.00- 40.00
Erythrocyte protoporphyrin	10.00- 15.00	Sodium (serum)	3.50- 5.00
		Tellurium	21.00- 45.00
Ethanol	8.00- 15.00	Thallium	18.00- 40.00
Fluoride (serum)	13.00- 20.00	Toluene	115.00
Gold	25.00- 35.00	Vanadium	21.00
Indium	20.00- 35.00	Xylene	115.00
Iodine (serum)	7.00- 10.00	Zinc	5.00- 22.00

*Prices depend on the quantities per order, the total annual order volume, and the method used for the test.

Serology is rarely performed in occupational medicine. Several of the respondents to the F&S survey, however, reported offering the VDRL test to detect venereal diseases.

The most targeted blood testing available to the occupational physician is that directed at measuring blood levels of certain chemical susbtances. Such tests provide a biological monitoring method to evaluate the degree of exposure of individual employees to harmful substances. The new standard for lead exposure, for instance, requires that biological monitoring of blood lead levels of exposed workers be undertaken to identify those who have been exposed to dangerous lead levels before any disease states become evident. Similar blood tests are also available for numerous toxic substances, as listed in Table 27.

The most common techniques to monitor the amount of lead in the human body are atomic absorption, anodic stryping voltammetry, and zinc protoporphyrin. The CDC has been recommending the latter, which is performed by the use of a fluorometer that also indicates iron deficiency anemias. Fluorometers

Table 28: Number and Percent of Plants and Employees in Plants Covered by Periodic Blood Tests for Employees

Code	Industry	Small (8-99)	Medium (100-500)	Large (Over 500)	Total
20	Food and kindred products	452 (3.5)	336 (11.3)	86 (21.3)	873 (5.4)
21	Tobacco products			15 (37.5)	15 (7.7)
22	Textile mill products	108 (4.0)	10 (2.0)	8 (21.6)	125 (3.9)
23	Apparel and other textile products	194 (1.5)	38 (1.6)		232 (1.5)
24	Lumber and wood products	141 (5.1)			141 (4.6)
25	Furniture and fixtures		8 (1.2)	10 (13.2)	18 (0.4)
26	Paper and allied products	30 (0.9)	130 (9.2)	39 (18.9)	198 (4.1)
27	Printing and publishing	67 (0.6)	27 (1.8)		93 (0.7)
28	Chemicals and allied products	914 (17.1)	118 (12.8)	164 (35.1)	1,197 (17.8)
29	Petroleum and coal products	16 (2.3)	59 (25.1)	34 (54.0)	109 (11.0)
30	Rubber and miscellaneous plastics	880 (19.5)	59 (6.0)	55 (37.2)	994 (17.6)
31	Leather and leather products				
32	Stone, clay and glass products	658 (10.3)	179 (12.5)	31 (21.7)	868 (10.9)
33	Primary metals	105 (2.8)	182 (19.7)	157 (43.3)	444 (8.8)
34	Fabricated metals	487 (2.9)	197 (7.5)	82 (20.3)	766 (3.9)
35	Machinery, except electrical	31 (0.3)	94 (5.1)	148 (25.6)	273 (1.9)
36	Electric and electronic equipment	160 (5.2)	66 (4.4)	139 (30.0)	365 (7.2)
37	Transportation equipment	35 (1.4)	24 (3.9)	128 (34.5)	187 (5.4)
38	Instruments	20 (0.6)	31 (8.5)	2 (1.0)	53 (1.4)
39	Miscellaneous manufacturing		32 (4.4)	50 (52.6)	82 (1.4)

Table 28: continued

Employees in Plants (thousands)

Code	Industry	Small (8–99)	Medium (100–500)	Large (Over 500)	Total
20	Food and kindred products	24 (6.5)	98 (14.2)	63 (18.7)	186 (13.2)
21	Tobacco products	—	—	21 (32.1)	21 (26.1)
22	Textile mill products	2 (2.0)	2 (2.3)	7 (15.6)	11 (4.7)
23	Apparel and other textile products	12 (2.4)	11 (2.9)	—	23 (2.5)
24	Lumber and wood products	4 (4.9)	—	—	4 (2.5)
25	Furniture and fixtures	1 (1.2)	1 (1.2)	9 (16.8)	10 (3.6)
26	Paper and allied products	1 (1.2)	20 (7.7)	50 (28.0)	72 (12.6)
27	Printing and publishing	6 (1.7)	8 (2.5)	—	14 (1.1)
28	Chemicals and allied products	34 (17.6)	25 (13.0)	314 (54.2)	373 (38.7)
29	Petroleum and coal products	1 (4.3)	15 (28.1)	75 (61.8)	91 (46.7)
30	Rubber and miscellaneous plastics	14 (10.1)	20 (10.2)	125 (61.3)	159 (29.8)
31	Leather and leather products	—	—	—	—
32	Stone, clay and glass products	22 (12.4)	55 (17.9)	124 (58.2)	202 (28.8)
33	Primary metals	5 (4.4)	53 (24.0)	689 (68.6)	747 (55.4)
34	Fabricated metals	14 (3.1)	54 (10.5)	65 (16.9)	133 (9.9)
35	Machinery, except electrical	2 (0.7)	24 (6.6)	306 (34.1)	333 (21.6)
36	Electric and electronic equipment	6 (5.8)	16 (4.8)	667 (62.3)	688 (45.9)
37	Transportation equipment	2 (2.5)	5 (3.5)	496 (49.6)	503 (41.1)
38	Instruments	686 (0.8)	5 (7.5)	6 (2.5)	12 (3.1)
39	Miscellaneous manufacturing	—	10 (6.6)	53 (56.9)	63 (16.4)

SOURCE: NIOSH Occupational Hazard Survey, 1977.

are electro-optical instruments that directly measure zinc protoporphyrin in whole blood in ten seconds without sample preparation.

Free erythrocyte protoporphyrin (FEP) is also an excellent indicator of poisoning. FEP can be measured rapidly and precisely by a micromethod.

Attempts are being made to determine the effects of zinc and cadmium exposure on aminolevulinic acid dehydrase (ALAD) activity, aminolevulinic acid (ALA) excretion, and FEP concentration in lead intoxication to ensure that the current screening tests are not recording false negative results in lead intoxicated individuals exposed simultaneously to high levels of zinc or cadmium.

Nearly all laboratory tests are performed by outside providers, although very large plants often have some laboratory equipment in-house. For instance, 16 percent of the respondents to the F&S survey had some type of limited laboratory facility in the plant. Many companies whose workers are exposed to lead, for example, acquire fluorometers to perform blood tests on their employees to comply with the biological monitoring requirements of the OSHA standard.

Urinalysis

Urinalysis is a common screening procedure in industrial medicine. The NIOSH survey[42] estimates that in the mid 1970s 2.9 percent of all plants employing 14.4 percent of all workers offered periodic urine tests as a part of a medical screening procedure. Moreover, 22.1 percent of plants employing 500 or more workers per plant, representing 34.4 percent of all workers employed by such plants, provided periodic urine tests (see Table 18). In the manufacturing industries 4.8 percent of all plants, representing 24.6 percent of all workers, provided such tests. Moreover, 26.4 percent of all plants employing 500 or more workers per plant, representing 44.6 percent of workers employed by such plants, provided urine tests (see Table 30). Companies responding to the F&S survey reported a much higher usage of urine tests, with 78 percent of the facilities providing the service (see Table 17).

Urinalysis is recommended as a screening procedure for workers exposed to numerous OSHA-regulated substances, as shown in Table 26.

Urinalysis is used to detect diseases of the kidney and the urinary tract and for diabetes. The test procedures include such evaluations as albumin, glucose, bilirubin, acetone, and occult blood. Abnormal findings often indicate kidney disease, although they appear after the damage is significant. Also, these abnormalities can be associated with exposures to certain hazardous substances.

Urine evaluations are also used to detect trace metals in the system, which can aid in assessing the degree of worker exposure to hazardous materials. Such tests are listed in Table 29.

Table 29: Urine Tests Available to Detect Dangerous Exposures to Workplace Hazards

Tests	Price Range*	Tests	Price Range*
Aluminum	$40.00–$70.00	Magnesium	6.50– 22.00
Antimony	25.00– 45.00	Manganese	18.00– 40.00
Arsenic	15.00– 45.00	Mercury	15.00– 45.00
Benzidine	25.00– 30.00	Molybdenum	
Beryllium	21.00– 45.00	Nickel	18.00– 40.00
Bismuth	18.00– 45.00	Organophosphates	
Cadmium	10.00– 45.00	(pesticides)	21.00– 45.00
Calcium	4.50– 6.50	Phenol	18.00– 25.00
Carbon		Selenium	21.00– 45.00
Chromium	16.50– 60.00	Silver	21.00– 40.00
Cobalt	18.00– 30.00	Tellurium	21.00– 45.00
Copper	8.00– 22.00	Thallium	18.00– 40.00
Delta-amino-		Tin	21.00– 35.00
levulinic acid	15.00– 21.00	Toluene	115.00
Fluoride		Trichloroethylene	
Gold	15.00– 30.00	metabolites	
Herbicide screen		Vanadium	
Indium	20.00– 35.00	Xylene	115.00
Iron	7.50– 12.00	Zinc	10.00– 22.00
Lead	6.00– 18.00		

*Prices depend on the quantities per order volume and the method used for the test.

Cytology

Cytology is the examination of the cell for abnormal anatomy or for cellular changes, using gross or microscopic techniques. Cytology holds substantial promise as a method of screening for cancer or precancerous conditions. Unfortunately, the efficacy of cytology as a screening device has not been demonstrated conclusively in many types of cancer, with the exception of cervical cancer, where it has met with an unqualified success.

In pure occupational medicine applications only sputum and urinary cytology have been recommended for a very selected population exposed to OSHA-regulated substances. Other cytologic tests, such as genetic evaluations, are currently used experimentally to identify individuals with tendencies to develop certain diseases. Also, many preventive medicine programs sponsored by corporations include Pap smear cytologies to identify cervical cancer in women employees.

Table 30: Number and Percent of Plants and Employees in Plants Covered by Periodic Urine Tests for Employees

Code	Industry	Small (8–99)	Plants Medium (100–500)	Large (Over 500)	Total
20	Food and kindred products	353 (2.8)	290 (9.7)	107 (26.5)	749 (4.6)
21	Tobacco products	—	—	15 (37.5)	15 (7.7)
22	Textile mill products	108 (4.0)	10 (2.0)	8 (21.6)	125 (3.9)
23	Apparel and other textile products	194 (1.5)	38 (1.6)	—	232 (1.5)
24	Lumber and wood products	141 (5.1)	—	—	141 (4.6)
25	Furniture and fixtures	—	20 (2.9)	10 (13.2)	30 (0.6)
26	Paper and allied products	—	60 (4.3)	39 (18.9)	98 (2.0)
27	Printing and publishing	67 (0.6)	43 (2.9)	38 (10.3)	148 (1.1)
28	Chemicals and allied products	800 (14.9)	139 (15.1)	114 (24.4)	1,054 (15.6)
29	Petroleum and coal products	16 (2.3)	59 (25.1)	34 (54.0)	109 (11.0)
30	Rubber and miscellaneous plastics	853 (18.9)	67 (6.8)	55 (37.2)	975 (17.3)
31	Leather and leather products	—	—	—	—
32	Stone, clay and glass products	658 (10.3)	179 (12.5)	31 (21.7)	867 (10.9)
33	Primary metals	133 (3.5)	140 (15.2)	185 (51.0)	458 (9.1)
34	Fabricated metals	555 (3.3)	209 (7.9)	128 (31.7)	891 (4.5)
35	Machinery, except electrical	31 (0.3)	37 (2.0)	181 (31.3)	248 (1.7)
36	Electric and electronic equipment	133 (4.3)	118 (7.8)	140 (30.2)	390 (7.7)
37	Transportation equipment	—	16 (2.6)	72 (19.4)	88 (2.5)
38	Instruments	—	22 (6.0)	5 (2.5)	27 (0.7)
39	Miscellaneous manufacturing	—	32 (4.4)	44 (46.3)	76 (1.3)

Table 30: continued

Code	Industry	Small (8-99)	Employees in Plants (thousands) Medium (100-500)	Large (Over 500)	Total
20	Food and kindred products	22 (5.8)	81 (11.8)	77 (23.0)	180 (12.8)
21	Tobacco products	—	—	21 (32.1)	21 (26.1)
22	Textile mill products	2 (2.0)	2 (2.3)	7 (15.6)	11 (4.7)
23	Apparel and other textile products	12 (2.4)	11 (2.9)	—	23 (2.5)
24	Lumber and wood products	4 (4.9)	—	—	4 (2.5)
25	Furniture and fixtures	—	4 (3.6)	9 (16.8)	13 (4.6)
26	Paper and allied products	—	8 (3.2)	50 (28.0)	58 (10.3)
27	Printing and publishing	6 (1.7)	9 (2.9)	58 (10.1)	73 (5.9)
28	Chemicals and allied products	26 (13.1)	31 (16.2)	282 (48.9)	340 (35.2)
29	Petroleum and coal products	875 (4.3)	15 (28.1)	75 (61.8)	91 (46.7)
30	Rubber and miscellaneous plastics	13 (9.6)	23 (11.9)	125 (61.3)	161 (30.2)
31	Leather and leather products	—	—	—	—
32	Stone, clay and glass products	22 (12.4)	55 (17.9)	124 (58.2)	202 (28.8)
33	Primary metals	7 (5.7)	44 (19.8)	848 (84.4)	899 (66.7)
34	Fabricated metals	18 (4.1)	63 (12.3)	108 (28.0)	190 (14.1)
35	Machinery, except electrical	2 (0.7)	8 (2.3)	349 (38.9)	359 (23.4)
36	Electric and electronic equipment	4 (3.7)	25 (7.6)	657 (61.4)	686 (45.7)
37	Transportation equipment	—	2 (1.3)	357 (35.7)	359 (29.3)
38	Instruments	—	4 (6.1)	10 (4.3)	14 (3.7)
39	Miscellaneous manufacturing	—	10 (6.6)	40 (42.8)	50 (13.0)

SOURCE: NIOSH Occupational Hazard Survey, 1977.

Screening for cancer with cytology is controversial for many applications, as will be discussed below. Also, there is considerable criticism regarding the quality of cytology testing. Currently, there are approximately 3000 registered cytology technicians in the United States.

Cancer cytology is an expensive testing technique. Most automated equipment, such as image analyzers and flow cytometers, are either too expensive or have limited diagnostic capabilities. Considerable developmental effort is necessary to bring these techniques to the stage where they can be routinely applied for mass screening.

Sputum Cytology. Sputum cytology is used as a screening procedure for the early detection of pulmonary disorders, particularly lung cancer.

Inflammation of the pulmonary system can be detected by measuring its cellularity. Increased cellularity (alveolar phagocytes, neutrophils, and lymphocytes) after exposure to heavy air pollution precedes the appearance of symptoms and can thus be used as an early marker of impending lung diseases.

As presented in chapter 4, sputum cytology for the early detection of lung cancer has not been found to be effective as a screening technique and it has been recommended that it not be used in screening industrial populations at risk.

Other sources, however, recommended sputum cytology and claim it is 90 percent accurate and can detect lung cancer well before it becomes visible on an x-ray film. Since cytology is a noninvasive procedure that does not expose the patient to any harmful agents, it is a very attractive test.

Only a small number of contributors (10.3 percent) to the F&S survey include sputum cytology in their screening program, as can be seen in Table 17. Unfortunately, NIOSH did not include this test in its survey and so any comparisons are impossible. More detailed information as to the industries reporting use of this test can be found in chapter 9.

Urinary Cytology. Urinary cytology is used to pinpoint cell changes from normal to cancerous at a very early stage in the development of cancer and before it can be detected by urinalysis (blood in urine). Urine cytology is recommended in the screening of workers exposed to substances known to cause kidney adenosarcoma. This cancer, if diagnosed early, has an excellent prognosis but such diagnosis is rarely possible without urine cytology. Urine cytology is also used in screening for bladder cancer.

Cytogenetics. Cytogenetics aims to identify genetic traits that when triggered by environmental factors produce selected human diseases, such as certain forms of cancer, diabetes, and multiple sclerosis. Cytogenetics examines the cell and genetic structure of a biostatistical sample of blood leukocytes. Cell studies seek to identify somatic cell damage that can be an early warning for impending serious disease.

Cytogenetic evaluations also identify the mutagenic and teratogenic effects of toxic substances. Tests carried out among workers exposed to vinyl chloride and other industrial substances have shown increased levels of chromosome breakage and other abnormalities.

Cytogenetic testing is an expensive procedure. Automatic techniques have not yet been developed to the point of practical routine use.

Cytogenetic evaluations are being carried out on a larger scale in European countries, such as Norway (vinyl chloride exposure) and Italy (benzene exposure). Cytogenetics could provide an early warning system before disease appears.

Other Laboratory Tests

In addition to the tests reported in previous subsections there are several other clinical laboratory procedures that are used by the occupational medicine field for special situations or on a very selective basis.

Hair Analysis. It has been suggested that trace metal analysis of the hair of exposed individuals could provide a valuable tool in the diagnosis of dangerous exposure before the advent of disease symptoms. Analysis of hair is not currently considered a practical clinical procedure because of the high level of contamination present in the hair due to external agents (shampoos, dyes, environmental contaminants), which diminishes the accuracy of laboratory tests. Nevertheless, many laboratories offer hair analyses, particularly for trace metals, such as lead, arsenic, copper, thallium, and zinc.

Tissue Analysis. Several metals and other hazardous substances can be biologically monitored by tissue analysis. Such substances include arsenic, lead, cadmium, copper, zinc, pesticides, and PCBs. Such tests tend to be expensive and are not practical for mass screening.

Reproductive Function Evaluations. Many industrial substances are known to affect reproductive function in males, as shown in Table 6. One way to diagnose the effect of such agents is to perform semen analysis to evaluate testicular function. A minimum of three valid semen analyses must be performed to obtain an accurate determination of sperm count. Sperm density is determined by the use of a white cell pipette and a hemocytometer chamber. The Papanicolaou technique is used to obtain a morphological evaluation. Other recorded characteristics include sperm agglutination, pyospermia, hyperviscosity, and pH. Samples are also evaluated for sperm viability (percent of viable sperm moving at the time of examination) and mobility. Serum determinations to be performed using radioimmunoassay techniques include: serum follicle stimulating hormone (FSH), serum luteinizing hormone (LH), and testosterone.

Liver Function Evaluations. Many industrial substances are toxic to the liver as listed in Table 9. Also, signs of abnormal liver function do not become apparent until after serious damage has taken place. However, NIOSH recommends liver function evaluations for workers exposed to Kepone and vinyl chloride. Tests commonly used for such evaluations include bile acids, total bilirubin, alkaline phosphatase, SGPT, lactic dehydrogenase (LDH), serum proteins, SGOT, and GGTP.

Hypersusceptibility Testing. There are individuals who have hereditary traits that make them exceptionally sensitive to certain substances. Exposure to such substances can cause severe reactions or can result in serious chronic disorders. It is therefore possible to test prospective employees during the preplacement examination for any susceptibilities that could result in serious illness because of the nature of the employment sought.

One technique to identify a hereditary deficiency that predisposes individuals to hypersensitivity to lung disease is the serum alpha$_1$-antitrypsin test. Also, the glucose-6-phosphate dehydrogenase test identifies individuals who have a hypersusceptibility to develop hemolytic disorders if exposed to hazardous agents. Currently, the most promising means of identifying individuals with susceptibility to certain diseases is the understanding of the HLA (histocompatibility) system. Such diverse disorders as psoriasis, arthritis, chronic hepatitis, asthma, and diabetes have been traced to certain HLA antigen combinations.

It is forecast that hypersusceptibility screening will become a very important screening modality in industrial occupational medicine programs. Already, large employers like DuPont and Dow Chemical offer some type of hypersusceptibility testing to those employed at high-risk occupations who volunteer to have the test performed.

OPHTHALMOLOGICAL SCREENING

Ophthalmological screening is a commonly used procedure in occupational medicine. Regulations require that ophthalmological tests be performed on certain classes of workers, such as drivers and pilots. Also many industries provide such ophthalmological tests to insure the safety of the worker and his co-workers.

Most commonly performed tests are those designed to measure visual acuity. More sophisticated tests involve viewing the eye by the use of the ophthalmoscope and the use of tonometry to diagnose glaucoma. Glaucoma is a serious eye disorder that, if undetected and untreated, results in blindness. The disease mostly affects those older than 40 years, but it can affect a person at any age. Estimates place Americans with glaucoma at 5-10 million people. Probably one half of those having the disorder are unaware of its presence. Glaucoma can be diagnosed by tonometry, which measures intraocular pressure noninvasively.

As discussed before, many substances are irritating to the eyes but few cause permanent damage and hardly any guidelines exist for ophthalmological evaluation in industrial medicine. One occupational group that must undergo eye tests periodically are truck and bus drivers.

The NIOSH survey estimates that 5.9 percent of all plants provided ophthalmological screening to 22.3 percent of all employees. Moreover, 33.7 percent of all plants with 500 or more employees offered this screening procedure. This is basically in agreement with the F&S survey results, showing that 31.9 percent of all companies offered this test periodically. Also, 38.6 percent of the respondents had some type of ophthalmological screening equipment in their medical departments and 2.4 percent said they intend to buy them in the future. The higher percentage of owners to providers reflects the inclusion of service companies in the total.

In addition 7.3 percent of the respondents owned tonometry devices (see Table 19) and 1.2 percent intended to buy them in the future (see Table 20).

According to NIOSH estimates, ophthalmological screening was more common among the manufacturing companies, with 7.4 percent of plants representing 33 percent of all workers offering the service. Results by individual industries within the general group are shown in Table 31.

Companies whose products were mentioned most often by the respondents include: Bausch & Lomb (6.2 percent), Titmus Optical (2.9 percent), American Optical (1 percent), and Keystone (1 percent).

OTHER TESTS

There are several other tests used in occupational medicine. These include neurological evaluations, tests of strength and stamina, body posture and joint flexibility, proctoscopy and sigmoidoscopy, breath testing, dental examinations, and radiation exposure tests.

Many agents cause neurological disorders, as shown in Table 7. Also, neurological problems might be early indicators of toxicity. One test to evaluate neurological status is the saccade velocity measurement (rapid eye movement) technique. The equipment for this test consists of a screen and a source projecting a pinpoint light on the screen. The subject's head is immobilized in a brace. The light appears at different parts of the screen in a random pattern. The subject's eye movements are measured using three electrodes attached to the forehead and temples. These electrodes pick up electrical signals created by the eye movement. These signals can then be analyzed by computer. This technique obtains five test indexes: maximum eye speed, accuracy of focus, delay time in shifting focus, smooth pursuit of a moving object, and maximum attainable eye velocity.

It is often also necessary to measure occupationally induced sensory loss in the fingertips (Raynaud's syndrome) of workmen exposed to vibration through

Table 31: Number and Percent of Plants and Employees in Plants Covered by Periodic Ophthalmological Examinations for Employees

Code	Industry	Small (8–99)	Plants Medium (100–500)	Large (Over 500)	Total
20	Food and kindred products	755 (5.9)	456 (15.3)	205 (50.7)	1,416 (8.8)
21	Tobacco products	—	11 (32.4)	15 (37.5)	26 (13.3)
22	Textile mill products	134 (5.0)	36 (7.3)	8 (21.6)	177 (5.5)
23	Apparel and other textile products	383 (2.9)	91 (3.9)	—	474 (3.0)
24	Lumber and wood products	233 (8.4)	10 (3.6)	13 (37.1)	256 (8.3)
25	Furniture and fixtures	37 (1.0)	57 (8.4)	43 (56.6)	136 (2.9)
26	Paper and allied products	85 (2.6)	190 (13.5)	62 (30.1)	337 (6.9)
27	Printing and publishing	67 (0.6)	58 (3.9)	69 (18.7)	194 (1.4)
28	Chemicals and allied products	450 (8.4)	204 (22.1)	210 (45.0)	864 (12.8)
29	Petroleum and coal products	71 (10.2)	79 (33.6)	56 (88.9)	207 (20.8)
30	Rubber and miscellaneous plastics	1,202 (26.6)	72 (7.3)	14 (9.5)	1,289 (22.9)
31	Leather and leather products	—	—	3 (8.8)	3 (0.2)
32	Stone, clay and glass products	882 (13.8)	272 (19.0)	31 (21.7)	1,185 (14.9)
33	Primary metals	129 (3.4)	182 (19.7)	209 (57.6)	520 (10.3)
34	Fabricated metals	1,461 (8.8)	477 (18.1)	129 (31.9)	2,067 (10.5)
35	Machinery, except electrical	130 (1.1)	124 (6.7)	276 (47.8)	531 (3.7)
36	Electric and electronic equipment	45 (1.5)	52 (3.4)	160 (34.6)	257 (5.1)
37	Transportation equipment	65 (2.6)	53 (8.6)	188 (50.7)	306 (8.9)
38	Instruments	—	54 (14.8)	14 (7.1)	69 (1.8)
39	Miscellaneous manufacturing	66 (1.3)	29 (4.0)	14 (14.7)	109 (1.9)

Table 31: continued

Code	Industry	Small (8-99)	Employees in Plants (thousands) Medium (100-500)	Large (Over 500)	Total
20	Food and kindred products	35 (9.2)	115 (16.7)	176 (52.2)	326 (23.2)
21	Tobacco products	—	3 (32.6)	21 (32.1)	24 (30.4)
22	Textile mill products	3 (3.2)	12 (12.4)	7 (15.6)	22 (9.4)
23	Apparel and other textile products	20 (3.9)	20 (5.2)	—	39 (4.3)
24	Lumber and wood products	6 (7.1)	2 (5.9)	12 (44.7)	21 (12.9)
25	Furniture and fixtures	1 (0.9)	13 (10.4)	32 (60.4)	47 (15.8)
26	Paper and allied products	4 (3.1)	43 (16.2)	80 (44.9)	127 (22.3)
27	Printing and publishing	6 (1.7)	22 (7.0)	118 (20.4)	146 (11.8)
28	Chemicals and allied products	19 (9.6)	45 (23.5)	352 (60.9)	416 (43.1)
29	Petroleum and coal products	4 (17.9)	23 (43.0)	118 (96.8)	145 (73.9)
30	Rubber and miscellaneous plastics	17 (12.1)	20 (10.8)	83 (40.4)	120 (22.5)
31	Leather and leather products	—	—	6 (25.1)	6 (4.1)
32	Stone, clay and glass products	27 (15.3)	64 (20.8)	124 (58.2)	216 (30.8)
33	Primary metals	6 (5.3)	54 (24.2)	864 (86.0)	924 (68.6)
34	Fabricated metals	57 (12.9)	120 (23.3)	129 (33.6)	307 (22.8)
35	Machinery, except electrical	8 (3.0)	28 (7.6)	610 (67.9)	647 (42.0)
36	Electric and electronic equipment	3 (3.6)	13 (4.0)	772 (72.1)	789 (52.6)
37	Transportation equipment	4 (5.4)	12 (8.2)	590 (59.0)	606 (49.6)
38	Instruments	—	12 (16.6)	47 (20.9)	59 (15.3)
39	Miscellaneous manufacturing	1 (0.7)	4 (2.8)	21 (23.0)	27 (7.0)

SOURCE: NIOSH Occupational Hazards Survey.

the operation of hand-held tools. Equipment devised to measure sensory loss (aesthesiometers) evaluate depth-sense perception and two-point discrimination.

Aesthesiometers are also used to evaluate peripheral circulation. Another technique used in occupational medicine to assess the status of the vascular bed of the limbs is multifinger photocell plethysmography. This technique records changes in the peripheral blood volume and is used to diagnose Raynaud's disease. A version of this instrument has been developed by NIOSH researchers. It consists of a power supply and six fiberoptic bundles. Each bundle transmits light to a finger inserter made of an acetal resin material. Each finger is placed between a fiberoptic bundle and a cadmium sulfide photodetector. After the photodetector output is amplified and conditioned, it is simultaneously presented to a tape recorder and to a strip-chart recorder for visual display and a permanent record.

Neurobehavioral changes might also be the earliest indicators of subclinical lead intoxication. Behavioral indicators, such as speed and quantitative characteristics of eye movement as detected by electro-oculographic methods, can serve as an effective screening tool for lead exposure monitoring.

Body posture and joint flexibility are tested using premeasured charts.

Radiation exposure levels can be measured by whole body scans. Such tests are now being performed on nuclear workers and residents of the area around Three Mile Island to assess the long-term effects of radiation exposure. The program sponsored by DHHS is expected to study the effects of the accidental radiation leak on the nearby population in general, and pregnant women and plant workers in particular.

Proctoscopy and sigmoidoscopy is mostly used in executive examinations. The test is criticized as inappropriate in screening asymptomatic individuals.

Breath analysis is a useful tool in evaluating exposure to harmful levels of toxic gases. Kits are available to measure carbon monoxide content in the blood by measuring its content in breath. Such tests cost about $5.00. Similar kits exist for the measurement of alcohol in breath.

COMPUTERS

Computers will undoubtedly become a very important tool in occupational medicine. Plants employing hundreds of workers exposed to hazardous materials in one location and large corporations employing thousands of such workers in several locations will all eventually turn to the computer for both health information storage and updating, as well as for conducting epidemiological studies and identifying problem areas within each plant.

Applications of the computer in occupational medicine can be described as follows:

> storage of health data (automated medical histories, automated insertion of health data arriving from various sources),

updating of health data,
automated identification of abnormal findings,
correlation of abnormal findings with work environment characteristics to isolate potential exposure hazards, and
development of epidemiological studies (type, duration, and level of exposure of employees correlated with their health status, personal habits, and age).

Naturally, use of a computer is only practical and cost effective when the testing volume is very large. Facilities with 500 workers or more, which manufacture or use OSHA-regulated substances and therefore are required to screen workers periodically would need the services of a computer for data storage and processing.

Among the respondents to the F&S survey 7.8 percent said that they were evaluating computer products for future use.

MULTIPHASIC SCREENING INSTALLATIONS

The definition of a multiphasic screening installation is somewhat difficult to arrive at because of the variety of testing combinations that qualify. For the purpose of this study, we will assume that a complete installation would include equipment capable for performing all the tests listed in Table 18 (including EKG devices) with the exception of sophisticated clinical laboratory instrumentation, the installation of which is rarely justified in the case of low volume testing. A multiphasic screening facility of this nature will probably cost a company upward of $100,000 and would be economically justified only in a small percent of United States plants, but should represent an excellent investment for companies contracting their services to industry.

Multiphasic screening installations with the help of fully automated equipment and data processing systems can be highly efficient, often capable of screening up to 25 workers per day. Such an installation, used by the Dow Chemical Company, is capable of screening more than 6500 workers per year. Set ups using less automation are not as efficient.

When questioned as to the benefit and cost effectiveness of a multiphasic screening installation, the respondents to the F&S survey were generally against it (51.4 percent) with only 24.1 percent giving an affirmative answer. Another 9.5 percent (some of them hospitals) said they already had a multiphasic installation in operation. Selected comments made by the respondents follow:

> MP screening is too inclusive, requires considerable M.D. time, questionable positives have to be checked out and it is too expensive.
> We have run such an in-house program but the return was not worth the cost and time invested.
> Predesigned units are seldom inexpensive; screening must be designed for each plant on an individual basis.
> MP screening is only practical in plants with over 600 workers.

I believe in one-to-one relationship between employees and health professionals.

An MP installation could reduce the duration of a medical examination and serve as a focal point.

There is no sense in paying for tests that are not relevant. This gives one a false sense of security.

I am not sold on multiphasic screening as a routine program.

We feel MP is both beneficial and cost-effective.

Screening for hypertension alone has increased disability payments by 25 percent and also increased casual absenteeism.

Follow-up on random results is enormously costly in administrative as well as direct costs.

Tests must be agent-specific; MP is not appropriate.

MP screening would not be acceptable to the majority of the employees.

We tried MP once but were not happy with its "assembly-line" operation.

9
The Occupational Medicine Marketplace

The marketplace in the occupational medicine field is highly diverse and highly fragmented. It is a product of the 1970s and probably represents the most significant single effort to test the concept of preventive medicine through the use of some type of multiphasic screening.

In spite of the size and the diversity of the market a standardization of testing is evolving that makes this marketplace easier to analyze. As we have seen in chapter 8, there is a battery of tests considered relevant in a multiphasic testing program and those are performed routinely with slight modifications. Also, additional tests mandated by NIOSH and OSHA recommendations often augment this regimen to provide targeted screening techniques designed to safeguard the health of individuals who are exposed to specific hazardous substances or circumstances.

Although the screening philosophy and the testing regimens seem to become well accepted by industry at large, it is nearly impossible to obtain a clear picture of the degree of testing, its costs and methodology. NIOSH conducted a study[42] in the mid 1970s by surveying thousands of plants and using the data to estimate the penetration of certain types of medical screening techniques in industry. We have combined the results of the NIOSH survey with these obtained from the F&S survey to estimate the degree of medical surveillance provided by industry and to arrive at market figures to be presented later in this section.

THE MARKET

The size of the potential market is extremely large. The current work force in the United States exceeds 85 million people employed by more than five million businesses. However, the majority (87 percent) of these businesses employ fewer than 25 workers. It is estimated that of the 85 million workers 21 million are exposed to OSHA-regulated substances and about 880,000 are exposed to the carcinogens currently regulated by OSHA. Approximately 390,000 cases of occupationally induced disease and 100,000 deaths occur annually.

Present coverage of workers by organized occupational and safety services is judged to be inadequate. A NIOSH survey carried out between 1972 and 1974 involving 4636 workplaces, showed that only 31 percent of the plants covering 24 percent of the employees had industrial hygiene services and 4 percent of the plants (covering 31.5 percent of all workers) had formally established health units. Fewer than 2 percent of the employees of small businesses had access to industry health and safety services.

NIOSH also estimates that in 1974, 13,192,350 workers exposed to workplace hazards were employed by plants that did not offer any type of medical surveillance, as shown in Table 32.

Also, the cost of controlling the occupational environment to protect the worker could be substantial, perhaps staggering. A study conducted by the Foster D. Snell division of Booz Allen & Hamilton estimated that average annual costs of regulating potential carcinogens alone could range from $6 to $36 billion if all of the 2500 substances presently suspected of being carcinogens come under Category 1 regulations and current techniques are applied. Naturally, the latter is unlikely, but there is no question that worker protection will not be inexpensive.

In order to take a closer look into this marketplace it is necessary to obtain a profile of industry. Tables 33-35 summarize the market in terms of plants (by size) and total employees (by size of plant). In this section, concentration will be centered on two major industry segments: the manufacturing industries and the services sector. Other areas, such as agricultural services, forestry and fisheries, mining, and contract construction, are haphazardly regulated and dominated by small firms that do not have the resources to implement a health screening program.

A statistical analysis by industry, plant size, and geographical location of the respondents to the survey are given in Tables 36-40.

A discussion of the survey results in the manufacturing and service sectors follows. Comparisons are also made between the F&S results and estimates produced by NIOSH after it conducted a large-scale survey of all industries in the 1972-1974 period.

Table 32: Estimated Number of People by Industry Exposed to Hazards in Facilities that Do Not Provide Medical Examinations of Any Type

SIC Code	Industry	Total Estimate	Full-Time Estimate
	All industries	13,192,350	3,002,933
	Agricultural services, forestry, fisheries	64,016	9,112
	Mining (oil and gas)	15,008	4,109
	Contract construction	1,834,295	217,290
	Manufacturing	4,492,934	1,642,747
19	Ordnance and accessories	9,156	4,320
20	Food and kindred products	467,514	225,766
21	Tobacco manufacturers	10,592	9,540
22	Textile mill products	103,097	56,518
23	Apparel and other textile products	531,836	181,470
24	Lumber and wood products	81,259	42,531
25	Furniture and fixtures	156,000	56,511
26	Paper and allied products	216,588	99,030
27	Printing and publishing	366,497	91,528
28	Chemicals and allied products	159,661	30,423
29	Petroleum and coal products	24,881	6,413
30	Rubber and plastics products	208,655	120,254
31	Leather and leather products	93,815	35,200
32	Stone, clay and glass products	228,094	93,033
33	Primary metal industries	185,686	98,063
34	Fabricated metal products	557,116	190,695
35	Machinery, except electrical	386,229	87,194
36	Electrical equipment and supplies	250,324	69,822
37	Transportation equipment	166,323	63,125
38	Instruments and related products	97,920	14,919
39	Miscellaneous manufacturing industries	191,692	66,392
	Transportation and other public utilities	354,633	21,301
	Wholesale and retail trade	4,101,097	852,950
	Finance, insurance and real estate	406,178	12,267
	Services	1,924,189	243,156

SOURCE: National Occupational Hazard Survey, Vol. III, NIOSH, HEW, 1977.

Table 33: Number of Establishments and Total Employees by Industry Groups

Industry	No. of Establishments	No. of Employees
Manufacturing	312,662	18,032,300
Construction	920,806	4,145,800
Mining	25,269	595,100
Total	1,258,737	22,773,200

SOURCE: Annual Survey of Manufacturers, Industry Profiles, Department of Commerce, Bureau of the Census, June 1978.

Table 34: Number of Establishments by Industry and Special Features

Industry	No. of Establishments
Manufacturing, operating establishments with 20 or more employees	114,195
Mining, establishments with 20 employees or more	5,312
Construction, establishments with payroll	437,941
Total	557,448

SOURCE: Annual Survey of Manufacturers, Industry Profiles, Department of Commerce, Bureau of the Census, June 1978.

Table 35: Number of Plants and Employees in Plants in the Services Sector

Service	Plants Small (8-99)	Plants Medium (100-500)	Plants Large (Over 500)	Plants Total	Employees in Plants (thousands) Small (8-99)	Employees in Plants (thousands) Medium (100-500)	Employees in Plants (thousands) Large (Over 500)	Employees in Plants (thousands) Total
Transportation and other utilities	30,528	5,056	706	36,289	855.1	926.1	1,530	3,311.3
Wholesale and retail trade	226,434	13,675	1,244	281,353	5,432.7	2,319.3	1,531.8	9,283.8
Finance, insurance and real estate	48,622	3,615	230	52,467	1,085.7	634.1	226.5	1,946.3
Services, other	143,489	9,147	1,737	154,374	2,926.6	1,432.2	1,444.6	5,803.4

SOURCE: NIOSH Occupational Hazards Survey, Vol. 3, 1977.

Table 36: Industry Distribution of Survey Respondents — Manufacturing, Mining, and Construction

Industry	No. of Facilities	No. of Workers Supervised
Chemicals, pharmaceuticals, rubber, and allied products (SIC #28 and 30)	58	672,538
Electrical and electronic machinery and scientific instruments (SIC #36 and 38)	39	426,205
Machinery, except electrical (SIC #35)	31	95,808
Primary metals and stone, clay, and concrete (SIC #32 and 33)	31	142,083
Transportation equipment (SIC #37)	29	1,132,455
Petroleum and coal products (SIC #29)	12	124,560
Fabricated metals (SIC #34)	12	25,080
Paper, wood and allied (SIC #26)	10	80,900
Food and tobacco (SIC #20 and 21)	8	13,100
Textiles and furniture (SIC #25 and 22)	7	132,300
Consumer goods	6	108,800
Mining and construction	6	50,550
Nuclear	5	21,900
Printing and publishing (SIC #27)	2	2,700
Total	256	3,028,979

SOURCE: F&S Survey. Note: Questionnaires that arrived after the cut-off date were processed only within the individual industry category later in this section. Therefore, the totals do not correspond exactly.

Table 37: Industry Distribution of Survey Respondents—
Utilities, Financial, and Other Services

Types of Service	No. of Facilities	No. of Workers Supervised
Utilities	35	536,500
Telecommunications (SIC #48)	20	342,800
Energy (SIC #49)	8	35,700
Transportation (SIC #40, 44 and 45)	7	158,000
Financial (SIC #60 and 63)	22	141,590
Business and other services	44	232,710
Health services (SIC #80)	23	64,360
Educational services (SIC #82)	13	63,150
Other services (SIC #54, 56, 73 and 79)	8	105,200
Government	18	246,954
Federal agencies and armed forces	10	121,474
Municipal governments	8	125,480
Total	119	1,157,754

SOURCE: F&S Survey.

Table 38: Geographic Distribution of Survey Respondents — Manufacturing, Mining, and Construction

Geographic Location	No. of Facilities Represented	No. of Workers Supervised
Region I	16	61,075
CT	7	31,625
ME	3	10,700
MA	4	14,250
NH	1	2,500
RI	1	2,000
Region II	31	467,210
NY	15	384,260
NJ	16	82,950
Region III	29	120,578
DE	2	4,300
MD	4	16,078
PA	14	68,900
VA	7	26,300
WV	2	5,000
Region IV	22	178,828
AL	3	5,000
FL	3	15,525
GA	1	4,000
KY	4	11,130
NC	6	100,448
SC	3	36,000
TN	2	6,725
Region V	77	1,483,886
IL	16	91,810
IN	11	19,800
MN	7	120,650
MI	14	1,027,966
OH	22	177,910
WI	7	45,750
Region VI	21	162,212
LA	1	900
OK	3	55,800
TX	17	105,512
Region VII	6	10,920
IA	1	450
MO	2	7,700
NE	3	2,770

Table 38: continued

Geographic Location	No. of Facilities Represented		No. of Workers Supervised	
Region VIII	5		12,500	
CO		3		5,000
SD		1		2,000
UT		1		5,500
Region IX	14		60,270	
CA		9		29,070
AZ		2		7,900
NV		2		22,700
HI		1		600
Region X	14		73,350	
ID		5		47,400
OR		5		5,200
WA		4		22,750
N/A	21		396,150	
Total	256		3,028,979	

Table 39: Geographic Distribution of Survey Respondents— Utilities, Financial, and Other Services

Geographic Location	No. of Facilities Represented		No. of Workers Supervised
Region I	9		50,800
CT		3	12,000
ME		1	5,000
MA		5	33,800
Region II	21		185,974
NY		12	99,000
NJ		9	86,974
Region III	19		80,535
DE		1	3,500
DC		5	54,000
MD		5	11,350
PA		4	8,325
VA		2	460
WV		2	2,900
Region IV	4		69,200
AL		1	60,000
GA		1	200
SC		1	5,000
TN		1	4,000
Region V	20		74,315
IL		5	18,950
IN		3	18,350
MN		4	10,700
OH		3	12,500
WI		5	13,815
Region VI	3		47,900
TX		3	47,900
Region VII	1		2,500
NE		1	2,500
Region VIII	4		20,800
CO		2	13,500
UT		2	7,300
Region IX	29		477,950
CA		21	444,550
AZ		5	23,100
HI		3	10,300
N/A		9	147,780
Total	119		1,157,754

Table 40: Distribution of Survey Respondents by Size of Establishment

No. of Employees	No. of Respondents	% of Total
Fewer than 99	1	.3
100-500	30	7.7
500-999	56	14.4
1000-2499	86	22.1
2500 and over	216	55.5
Total	389	100

Manufacturing

The single largest market component is the manufacturing industries group. Many manufacturing processes have come under OSHA scrutiny and workers in these industries are daily exposed to various OSHA-regulated substances. Also, the manufacturing industries are considered one of the most hazardous workplaces, as can be seen from Table 41.

Tables 42-45 illustrate the size of this industry and the number of workers involved. The NIOSH survey[42] estimates of the degree of availability of medical screening programs in the manufacturing industries are presented in Table 46. In 1973 NIOSH estimated that 1,642,747 workers in this industry were exposed full-time to hazardous substances in plants that had no medical surveillance programs of any type (see Table 32).

In this subsection a comparison can be made between the results of the NIOSH survey, representing 1973, data and the results of the F&S survey. Unfortunately, comparisons are only possible for large-sized plants (500 workers and over), since very few medium and small-sized plants responded to the F&S survey.

Table 41: Ranking of Hazardous Industries

	Annual Injury and Illness Rate (per 100 Workers)	Occupational Illness Incidence (% of Total)
Industry by Type		
Construction	16.0	
Manufacturing	13.0	75
Mining	11.0	
Transportation	9.4	
Agriculture	8.5	
Sales	7.3	25
Services	5.4	
Finance	2.2	
*Industry by Size**		
Small business, low risk	7.2	
Small business, high risk	8.6	
Large business, low risk	2.9	
Large business, high risk	13.1	

*Small businesses are those with fewer than 25 employees.

SOURCE: Bureau of Labor Statistics.

Table. Manufacturing Employment by Industry Type (1972, 1976, and 1978 Statistics)

SIC Code	Major Industry Group	No. of Employees of Operating Establishments (thousands)			No. of Production Workers (thousands)		
		1972	1976	1978	1972	1976	1978
20	Food and kindred products	1,569.3	1,538.8	1,546.8	1,085.3	1,066.4	1,097.7
21	Tobacco	66.3	64.8	59.1	57.4	54.8	49.1
22	Textile mill products	952.6	875.9	861.8	836.0	765.3	752.5
23	Apparel and other textile products	1,368.3	1,270.5	1,321.8	1,198.3	1,109.3	1,151.9
24	Lumber and wood products	691.0	628.5	723.2	600.9	543.2	618.6
25	Furniture and fixtures	462.0	425.7	481.0	384.1	351.9	396.5
26	Paper and allied products	633.4	614.9	638.6	498.9	477.3	491.8
27	Printing and publishing	1,056.5	1,085.8	1,144.8	637.7	629.3	651.9
28	Chemicals and allied products	836.5	850.9	903.4	525.0	519.9	549.6
29	Petroleum and coal products	139.5	144.4	148.2	98	100.2	103.1
30	Rubber and other plastic products	617.7	627.4	748.0	486.8	488.9	587.1
31	Leather and leather products	273.4	247.1	244.4	240.6	215.9	213.9
32	Stone, clay and glass products	623.2	598.9	639.3	492.5	473.8	509.4
33	Primary metals	1,142.8	1,106.0	1,149.4	922.8	874.8	920.5
34	Fabricated metal products	1,493.3	1,471.3	1,625.1	1,148.0	1,122.8	1,251.2
35	Machinery, except electrical	1,827.7	1,959.7	2,235.4	1,267.2	1,332.2	1,519.2
36	Electric and electronic equipment	1,661.3	1,578.4	1,863.0	1,160.2	1,080.4	1,284.6
37	Transportation equipment	1,719.0	1,667.7	1,865.7	1,246.0	1,205.6	1,364.5
38	Instruments	453.2	518.1	600.1	291.3	321.8	374.8
39	Miscellaneous manufacturing industries	445.6	410.1	447.0	349.8	317.4	343.1
	Total	18,032.4	17,684.9	20,508.9	13,526.8	13,051.2	14,231.0

SOURCE: Census of Manufacturers, Department of Commerce.

Table 43: Number of Manufacturing Establishments by Size*

SIC Code	Industry	20-99 1972	20-99 1977	100-249 1972	100-249 1977
20	Food and kindred products	8,421	7,237	2,611	2,424
21	Tobacco products	63	38	41	41
22	Textile mill products	2,331	2,108	1,082	1,018
23	Apparel	8,731	8,415	2,347	2,424
24	Lumber and wood products	5,239	5,481	1,295	1,224
25	Furniture and fixtures	2,561	2,500	708	690
26	Paper and allied products	2,202	2,276	1,194	1,185
27	Printing and publishing	6,795	7,236	1,158	1,258
28	Chemicals	3,003	3,087	758	812
29	Petroleum and coal products	456	496	149	150
30	Rubber and miscellaneous plastics	2,871	3,740	871	1,025
31	Leather and leather products	885	824	400	337
32	Stone, clay and glass products	4,035	3,965	822	803
33	Primary metals	2,207	2,248	863	934
34	Fabricated metal products	8,576	9,422	2,009	2,182
35	Machinery, except electrical	7,673	9,082	1,597	1,854
36	Electric and electronic equipment	3,198	3,468	1,212	1,436
37	Transportation equipment	2,140	2,091	664	685
38	Instruments	1,306	1,630	413	462
39	Miscellaneous	2,827	2,885	606	602
	Total	75,520	78,229	20,800	21,546

*Only establishments with 20 employees or more.
SOURCE: Census of Manufacturers, Department of Commerce.

Table 43: continued

No. of Establishments										
250-499		500-999		1000-2499		2500 or More		Total	
1972	1977	1972	1977	1972	1977	1972	1977	1972	1977
893	947	303	335	80	86	17	13	12,325	11,042
24	27	13	7	7	4	6	6	154	123
649	587	325	309	107	97	10	12	4,504	4,131
881	845	220	208	42	35	5	6	12,226	11,933
260	278	56	60	18	12	——	1	6,868	7,056
245	254	102	116	27	26	4	2	3,647	3,588
335	315	158	153	65	68	2	3	3,956	4,000
390	375	174	182	83	75	19	19	8,619	9,145
345	348	184	213	107	109	34	36	4,431	4,605
57	63	36	45	17	18	5	2	720	774
260	340	102	105	71	70	13	14	4,188	5,294
301	265	65	56	6	5	——	——	1,657	1,487
258	257	132	128	46	42	8	6	5,301	5,201
428	412	212	215	119	99	72	73	3,901	3,981
688	746	273	277	92	78	38	35	11,676	12,740
673	775	388	453	203	218	65	69	10,599	12,451
626	709	374	420	218	204	104	101	5,732	6,338
330	378	188	192	132	146	164	161	3,618	3,653
169	237	105	129	59	62	14	20	2,066	2,540
220	206	71	74	28	26	2	2	3,754	3,795
8,032	8,364	3,481	3,677	1,527	1,480	582	581	109,942	113,577

Table 44: Number of All Employees of the Manufacturing Industries by Size of Establishment*

		Total Employees (thousands)			
		20-99		100-249	
SIC Code	Industry	1972	1977	1972	1977
20	Food and kindred products	386.3	340.2	406.4	377.4
21	Tobacco products	2.8	1.9	6.7	15.7[†]
22	Textile mill products	112.5	100.7	173.2	160.8
23	Apparel	403.0	384.2	365.7	377.1
24	Lumber and wood products	232.6	241.4	195.8	183.0
25	Furniture and fixtures	115.1	113.7	195.6[†]	106.6
26	Paper and allied products	107.1	112.0	187.1	178.8
27	Printing and publishing	281.0	301.0	175.2	189.0
28	Chemicals	132.7	137.3	237.5[†]	125.2
29	Petroleum and coal products	19.9	21.4	24.2	24.6
30	Rubber and miscellaneous plastics	133.3	176.6	135.6	159.7
31	Leather and leather products	42.4	40.4	63.9	55.9
32	Stone, clay and glass products	165.3	163.5	124.7	122.4
33	Primary metals	103.9	107.6	137.9	148.8
34	Fabricated metals	371.7	407.8	311.0	335.1
35	Machinery, except electrical	318.4	380.2	245.4	287.8
36	Electric and electronic equipment	150.4	165.6	190.8	226.3
37	Transportation equipment	98.3	98.6	103.1	107.2
38	Instruments	58.1	73.2	64.3	71.4
39	Miscellaneous manufacturing	121.0	122.7	93.5	162.8[†]
	Total	3,355.6	3,490.0	3,232.0	3,415.6

*Only establishments with 20 employees or more.
[†]Includes figures for next larger category that follows; data are combined to avoid disclosing operations of individual companies.
SOURCE: Census of Manufacturers, Department of Commerce.

Table 44: continued

				Total Employees (thousands)					
250-499		500-999		1000-2499		2500 or More		Total	
1972	1977	1972	1977	1972	1977	1972	1977	1972	1977
309.9	330.4	317.8†	224.9	—	119.4	57.0	43.9	1,477.4	1,436.2
7.7	—	7.9	4.8	10.6	5.9	30.1	31.9	65.8	60.2
228.0	205.0	221.4	208.5	150.9	132.3	47.2	49.4	933.2	856.7
300.5	286.8	140.9	131.8	57.9	48.1	18.0	21.4	1,286.0	1,249.4
85.7	92.8	36.9	39.3	23.6	18.1†	—	—	574.6	574.6
—	87.5	67.3	75.8	37.5	44.5†	12.7	—	428.2	428.1
113.5	106.6	109.2	105.9	101.2†	99.3	—	8.7	618.1	611.3
132.6	128.6	119.6	123.9	192.6†	112.8	—	65.9	901.0	921.2
—	121.4	127.6	146.8	165.7	165.3	132.8	141.8	796.3	837.8
19.8	21.2	24.6	31.6	25.5	39.8†	17.2	—	131.2	138.6
89.5	113.5	70.5	69.4	105.0	108.5	53.1	54.4	587.0	682.1
107.1	93.6	41.6	36.1	9.4	8.0	—	—	264.4	234.0
89.7	89.0	91.7	90.7	61.8	57.7	23.0	17.6	556.2	540.9
49.9	142.2	147.0	146.5	179.6	142.2	404.4	404.5	1,122.7	1,091.8
237.1	255.1	183.1	187.6	134.7	115.6	141.5	126.1	1,379.1	1,427.3
238.5	270.0	268.6	317.2	298.8	325.2	292.7	311.2	1,662.4	1,891.6
220.0	266.8	259.4	293.8	323.2	305.1	480.4	440.0	1,624.2	1,697.6
16.4	132.1	130.9	133.1	199.0	221.2	1,043.5	1,044.9	1,691.2	1,737.1
58.4	84.5	70.6	89.0	91.1	90.4	89.6	125.3	432.1	533.8
75.6	—	97.3	49.5	—	44.7	—	—	387.4	379.7
285.2	2,827.1	2,370.0	2,506.2	2,248.6	2,204.1	2,926.8	2,887.0	16,918.2	17,330.0

Table 45: Number of Production Workers in the Manufacturing Industries by Size of Establishment*

		No. of Production Workers (thousands)			
		20-99		100-249	
SIC Code	Industry	1972	1977	1972	1977
20	Food and kindred products	251.5	228.6	267.9	255.6
21	Tobacco products	2.4	1.5	5.6	12.9†
22	Textile mill products	97.0	86.3	151.4	139.5
23	Apparel	353.3	332.2	324.3	330.1
24	Lumber and wood products	199.7	204.7	168.4	155.8
25	Furniture and fixtures	94.9	92.6	163.4†	87.4
26	Paper and allied products	85.5	87.4	146.3	137.1
27	Printing and publishing	183.9	191.1	109.4	114.5
28	Chemicals	80.4	82.7	151.1†	78.4
29	Petroleum and coal products	13.1	14.3	18.0	17.9
30	Rubber and miscellaneous plastics	107.7	140.5	109.3	127.7
31	Leather and leather products	36.9	34.6	56.3	49.1
32	Stone, clay and glass products	123.4	122.0	99.5	97.4
33	Primary metals	85.1	86.6	111.6	118.7
34	Fabricated metals	290.9	315.7	238.3	256.8
35	Machinery, except electrical	233.5	276.6	169.1	195.7
36	Electric and electronic equipment	109.5	120.8	141.5	164.5
37	Transportation equipment	77.9	77.1	81.4	82.8
38	Instruments	38.9	48.1	41.9	46.3
39	Miscellaneous manufacturing	96.1	95.2	75.1	126.9†
	Total	2,561.6	2,638.6	2,481.2	2,595.1

*Only establishments with 20 employees or more.

†Includes figures for the next larger category that follows; data are combined to avoid disclosing operations of individual companies.

SOURCE: Census of Manufacturers, Department of Commerce.

Table 45: continued

				No. of Production Workers (thousands)					
250-499		500-999		1000-2499		2500 or More		Total	
1972	1977	1972	1977	1972	1977	1972	1977	1972	1977
220.0	235.3	240.4†	170.8	—	90.6	40.7	31.3	1,020.5	1,012.2
6.2	—	7.1	4.1	9.3	5.1	26.4	26.4	57.0	50.0
200.6	174.5	193.7	183.0	133.6	115.2	43.7	44.4	820.0	742.9
264.1	252.3	122.5	112.1	49.5	40.2	14.6	16.5	1,128.3	1,083.4
74.5	80.1	31.6	33.4	20.0	15.2†	—	—	494.2	489.2
—	74.0	56.1	62.7	30.2	36.8†	10.5	—	355.1	353.5
89.8	84.0	87.0	83.7	78.0†	75.0	—	5.5	486.6	472.7
73.8	69.0	62.9	57.5	93.4†	50.7	—	25.3	523.4	508.1
—	77.4	81.2	93.9	106.8	103.0	80.4	81.7	499.9	517.1
13.4	14.8	17.6	20.9	18.2	27.4†	11.8	—	92.1	95.3
70.8	88.2	55.8	54.7	80.6	83.3	37.9	37.9	462.1	532.3
96.8	83.6	34.9	30.8	7.6	6.0	—	—	232.5	204.1
73.1	72.0	77.0	75.9	51.0	47.6	17.9	13.4	441.9	428.3
120.5	112.0	117.2	115.5	143.8	112.0	328.1	322.6	906.3	867.4
180.9	193.5	140.1	140.2	98.0	82.6	108.9	101.6	1,057.1	1,090.4
160.1	178.8	178.1	201.6	200.5	215.8	194.3	197.9	1,135.6	1,266.4
160.9	178.1	188.3	209.3	223.4	209.9	309.5	275.5	1,133.1	1,158.1
90.3	103.7	96.5	98.8	145.9	170.4	731.3	726.0	1,223.3	1,258.8
39.8	55.8	47.3	57.7	59.0	56.0	50.2	66.4	277.1	330.3
58.7	—	73.1†	37.3	—	31.2†	—	—	303.0	290.6
,143.5	2,127.1	1,785.8	1,843.9	1,629.1	1,574.0	2,048.1	1,972.4	12,649.4	12,751.1

Table 46: Summary of Number and Percent of Plants and Employees Covered by Special Medical Services—Manufacturing

	Manufacturing Industries				Employees (thousands)			
	Small (8-99)	Medium (100-500)	Large (Over 500)	Total	Small (8-99)	Medium (100-500)	Large (Over 500)	Total
Formally established health unit	2,562 (2.2)	5,711 (25.5)	3,677 (80.4)	11,950 (8.5)	126.7 (3.7)	1,502.8 (32.8)	6,418.5 (89.5)	8,048 (52.9)
Regularly record health information about new employees	63,437 (55.4)	19,043 (85.0)	4,524 (99.0)	87,005 (61.5)	2,163.4 (62.4)	4,061.3 (88.5)	7,138 (99.6)	13,362.7 (87.8)
Require preplacement physical examinations	20,681 (18.1)	11,921 (53.2)	3,992 (87.3)	36,594 (25.9)	777.5 (22.4)	2,718.4 (59.3)	6,714.3 (93.7)	10,210.2 (67.1)
Provide periodic medical examinations	12,143 (10.6)	6,268 (28.0)	2,700 (59.1)	21,111 (14.9)	450.2 (13.0)	1,479.5 (32.2)	5,398.4 (75.3)	7,328.1 (48.1)
Provide audiometric examinations	5,986 (5.2)	2,730 (12.2)	1,807 (39.5)	10,523 (7.4)	214.1 (6.2)	658.8 (14.4)	4,470.1 (62.4)	5,343 (35.1)
Provide periodic pulmonary function screening	3,595 (3.1)	1,281 (5.7)	995 (21.8)	5,870 (4.2)	140.5 (4.1)	327.8 (7.1)	3,116.9 (43.5)	3,585.2 (23.6)
Provide ophthalmological examinations	6,201 (5.4)	2,521 (11.3)	1,721 (37.7)	10,443 (7.4)	222.1 (6.4)	632.7 (13.8)	4,116.9 (58.1)	5,021.7 (33.0)
Provide x-ray examinations	8,172 (7.1)	4,280 (19.1)	1,865 (40.8)	14,318 (10.1)	299.3 (8.6)	1,019.1 (22.2)	4,149.3 (57.9)	5,467.7 (35.9)
Provide periodic urine tests	4,047 (3.5)	1,483 (6.6)	1,206 (26.4)	6,735 (4.8)	139.6 (4.0)	400.1 (8.7)	3,199.9 (44.6)	3,739.6 (24.6)
Provide periodic blood tests	4,303 (3.8)	1,596 (7.1)	1,164 (25.5)	7,063 (5.0)	151.4 (4.4)	426.7 (9.3)	3,086.1 (43.1)	3,664.2 (24.1)

Table 47: Number and Percent of Plants and Employees in Plants that Have a Formally Established Health Unit—Manufacturing

SIC Code	Industry	Plants Small (8–99)	Medium (100–500)	Large (Over 500)	Total
20	Food and kindred products	119 (0.9)	851 (28.5)	181 (44.8)	1,151 (7.1)
21	Tobacco products		28 (82.4)	40 (100)	67 (34.2)
22	Textile mill products	40 (1.5)	101 (20.4)	37 (100)	177 (5.5)
23	Apparel and other textile products	632 (4.8)	281 (12.1)	14 (31.8)	927 (6.0)
24	Lumber and wood products	50 (1.8)	29 (10.4)	22 (62.9)	101 (3.3)
25	Furniture and fixtures	27 (0.7)	148 (21.8)	51 (67.1)	226 (4.9)
26	Paper and allied products	64 (2.0)	342 (24.3)	206 (100)	611 (12.6)
27	Printing and publishing		141 (9.4)	307 (83.2)	448 (3.3)
28	Chemicals and allied products	210 (3.9)	391 (42.4)	371 (79.4)	972 (14.4)
29	Petroleum and coal products	55 (7.9)	93 (39.6)	63 (100)	211 (21.2)
30	Rubber and miscellaneous plastics	86 (1.9)	267 (27.2)	99 (66.9)	452 (8.0)
31	Leather and leather products	25 (2.1)	93 (21.1)	17 (50.0)	134 (8.1)
32	Stone, clay and glass products	121 (1.9)	351 (24.5)	128 (89.5)	599 (7.5)
33	Primary metals	511 (13.6)	382 (41.4)	363 (100)	1,256 (24.9)
34	Fabricated metals	346 (2.1)	738 (28.0)	329 (81.4)	1,412 (7.2)
35	Machinery, except electrical	81 (0.7)	540 (19.1)	423 (73.2)	1,043 (7.4)
36	Electric and electronic equipment	141 (4.6)	464 (30.7)	368 (79.5)	974 (19.2)
37	Transportation equipment		196 (31.7)	348 (93.8)	543 (15.7)
38	Instruments	24 (0.7)	102 (27.9)	192 (97.5)	319 (8.4)
39	Miscellaneous manufacturing	25 (0.5)	162 (22.3)	84 (88.4)	271 (4.7)

Table 47: continued

SIC Code	Industry	Small (8–99)	Medium (100–500)	Large (Over 500)	Total
20	Food and kindred products	7 (2.0)	239 (34.6)	186 (55.5)	433 (30.8)
21	Tobacco products		8 (80.1)	66 (100)	74 (91.8)
22	Textile mill products	1 (1.0)	27 (28.1)	43 (100)	71 (30.7)
23	Apparel and other textile products	32 (6.41)	55 (14.5)	19 (50.0)	106 (11.5)
24	Lumber and wood products	4 (4.9)	4 (8.1)	15 (55.3)	23 (14.2)
25	Furniture and fixtures	1 (1.1)	37 (29.0)	37 (69.4)	76 (25.7)
26	Paper and allied products	3 (2.6)	77 (29.1)	179 (100)	259 (45.4)
27	Printing and publishing		25 (8.2)	534 (92.5)	560 (45.2)
28	Chemicals and allied products	13 (6.9)	100 (52.2)	526 (90.8)	639 (66.1)
29	Petroleum and coal products	1 (6.1)	24 (44.5)	122 (100)	147 (75.2)
30	Rubber and miscellaneous plastics	3 (2.6)	65 (34.2)	178 (87.3)	248 (46.3)
31	Leather and leather products	1 (3.5)	25 (26.8)	16 (61.9)	42 (26.9)
32	Stone, clay and glass products	2 (7.5)	102 (33.4)	205 (96.1)	310 (44.2)
33	Primary metals	22 (18.4)	114 (51.2)	1,005 (100)	1,140 (84.6)
34	Fabricated metals	19 (4.2)	201 (39.0)	317 (82.4)	538 (39.8)
35	Machinery, except electrical	4 (1.7)	131 (35.6)	746 (82.9)	882 (57.3)
36	Electric and electronic equipment	6 (6.6)	133 (40.2)	905 (84.6)	1,045 (69.6)
37	Transportation equipment		56 (38.0)	984 (98.4)	1,040 (84.9)
38	Instruments	2 (1.9)	24 (33.9)	223 (98.4)	249 (64.6)
39	Miscellaneous manufacturing	2 (1.3)	48 (31.8)	87 (93.3)	137 (35.7)

SOURCE: NIOSH Occupational Hazards Survey, 1977.

Table 48: Number and Percent of Plants and Employees in Plants Covered by the Regular Recording of Health Information About New Employees

SIC Code	Industry	Small (8–99)	Medium (100–500)	Large (Over 500)	Total
20	Food and kindred products	7,425 (58.1)	2,851 (95.6)	404 (100.0)	10,680 (66.0)
21	Tobacco products	24 (19.7)	34 (100)	40 (100)	97 (49.5)
22	Textile mill products	1,488 (55.3)	353 (71.2)	37 (100)	1,877 (58.2)
23	Apparel and other textile products	2,586 (19.6)	922 (39.6)	44 (100)	3,552 (22.8)
24	Lumber and wood products	1,406 (50.6)	216 (77.4)	22 (62.9)	1,644 (53.2)
25	Furniture and fixtures	1,663 (43.1)	508 (74.7)	76 (100)	2,246 (48.6)
26	Paper and allied products	2,151 (66.2)	1,350 (95.9)	206 (100)	3,707 (76.3)
27	Printing and publishing	5,048 (43.0)	1,208 (80.7)	269 (100)	6,625 (48.7)
28	Chemicals and allied products	4,015 (75.0)	923 (100)	467 (100)	5,405 (80.2)
29	Petroleum and coal products	521 (75.0)	213 (90.6)	63 (100)	797 (80.3)
30	Rubber and miscellaneous plastics	3,576 (79.3)	867 (88.5)	138 (93.2)	4,580 (81.2)
31	Leather and leather products	544 (46.1)	220 (49.9)	24 (70.6)	788 (47.7)
32	Stone, clay and glass products	3,784 (59.3)	1,325 (92.3)	143 (100)	5,252 (66.0)
33	Primary metals	2,948 (78.5)	922 (100)	363 (100)	4,233 (84.0)
34	Fabricated metals	11,532 (69.6)	2,491 (94.4)	404 (100)	14,427 (73.6)
35	Machinery, except electrical	6,365 (54.1)	1,668 (89.9)	564 (97.6)	8,596 (60.6)
36	Electric and electronic equipment	2,439 (78.7)	1,459 (96.5)	463 (100)	4,360 (85.9)
37	Transportation equipment	1,849 (74.9)	575 (93.0)	371 (100)	2,796 (80.9)
38	Instruments	1,884 (58.0)	349 (95.4)	197 (100)	2,430 (63.7)
39	Miscellaneous manufacturing	2,161 (43.6)	557 (76.7)	95 (100)	2,814 (48.7)

Table 48: continued

SIC Code	Industry	Small (8-99)	Employees in Plants (thousands) Medium (100-500)	Large (Over 500)	Total
20	Food and kindred products	274 (72.8)	670 (96.8)	335 (100.0)	1,279 (91.1)
21	Tobacco products	1 (27.2)	10 (100)	65 (100)	77 (95.9)
22	Textile mill products	60 (64.9)	76 (78.5)	43 (100)	179 (77.1)
23	Apparel and other textile products	107 (21.4)	178 (47.0)	38 (100)	323 (35.1)
24	Lumber and wood products	53 (62.9)	41 (81.9)	15 (55.3)	109 (67.6)
25	Furniture and fixtures	57 (50.8)	97 (75.6)	54 (100)	208 (70.6)
26	Paper and allied products	93 (73.7)	254 (95.9)	179 (100)	526 (92.2)
27	Printing and publishing	193 (55.5)	261 (3.4)	578 (100)	1,032 (83.6)
28	Chemicals and allied products	147 (75.0)	191 (100)	579 (100)	917 (94.9)
29	Petroleum and coal products	17 (83.2)	48 (90.6)	122 (100)	187 (95.5)
30	Rubber and miscellaneous plastics	120 (86.9)	175 (91.2)	199 (97.4)	494 (92.5)
31	Leather and leather products	19 (51.2)	51 (55.9)	20 (81.0)	91 (58.8)
32	Stone, clay and glass products	124 (68.6)	289 (94.3)	214 (100)	626 (89.4)
33	Primary metals	107 (88.7)	222 (100)	1,005 (100)	1,334 (99.0)
34	Fabricated metals	342 (76.3)	493 (95.4)	385 (100)	1,220 (90.4)
35	Machinery, except electrical	180 (66.5)	343 (93.0)	891 (99.1)	1,414 (91.9)
36	Electric and electronic equipment	81 (81.4)	322 (97.3)	1,070 (100)	1,474 (98.2)
37	Transportation equipment	62 (80.9)	138 (94.3)	1,000 (100)	1,201 (98.1)
38	Instruments	54 (61.5)	67 (93.9)	227 (100)	348 (90.1)
39	Miscellaneous manufacturing	69 (49.6)	123 (81.7)	93 (100)	286 (74.5)

SOURCE: NIOSH Occupational Hazards Survey, 1977.

Table 49: Number and Percent of Plants and Employees in Plants Covered by Preplacement Physical Examinations of Employees

SIC Code	Industry	Plants Small (8-99)	Plants Medium (100-500)	Plants Large (Over 500)	Total
20	Food and kindred products	4,329 (33.9)	2,160 (72.5)	328 (81.2)	6,817 (42.2)
21	Tobacco products	5 (4.1)	22 (64.7)	9 (22.5)	37 (18.9)
22	Textile mill products	479 (17.8)	129 (26.0)	29 (78.4)	637 (19.8)
23	Apparel and other textile products	231 (1.8)	37 (1.6)	44 (100.0)	312 (2.0)
24	Lumber and wood products	593 (21.3)	119 (42.7)	25 (71.4)	737 (23.8)
25	Furniture and fixtures	203 (5.3)	247 (36.3)	68 (89.5)	518 (11.2)
26	Paper and allied products	841 (25.9)	1,102 (78.3)	206 (100.0)	2,149 (44.2)
27	Printing and publishing	444 (3.8)	413 (27.6)	279 (75.6)	1,136 (8.3)
28	Chemicals and allied products	2,252 (42.1)	661 (71.6)	416 (89.1)	3,329 (49.4)
29	Petroleum and coal products	229 (32.9)	225 (95.7)	63 (100.0)	517 (52.1)
30	Rubber and miscellaneous plastics	861 (19.1)	509 (51.9)	114 (77.0)	1,483 (26.3)
31	Leather and leather products	45 (3.8)	61 (13.8)	9 (26.5)	115 (7.0)
32	Stone, clay and glass products	1,507 (23.6)	1,145 (79.8)	128 (89.5)	2,780 (34.9)
33	Primary metals	1,618 (43.1)	787 (85.4)	348 (95.9)	2,753 (54.6)
34	Fabricated metals	3,439 (20.8)	1,850 (70.1)	404 (100.0)	5,694 (29.0)
35	Machinery, except electrical	1,545 (13.1)	1,151 (62.0)	539 (93.3)	3,235 (22.8)
36	Electric and electronic equipment	513 (16.6)	539 (35.6)	365 (78.8)	1,417 (27.9)
37	Transportation equipment	368 (14.9)	416 (67.3)	359 (96.8)	1,143 (33.1)
38	Instruments	431 (13.3)	154 (42.1)	192 (97.5)	777 (20.4)
39	Miscellaneous manufacturing	742 (15.0)	165 (22.7)	50 (52.6)	956 (16.6)

Table 49: continued

Employees in Plants (thousands)

SIC Code	Industry	Small (8-99)	Medium (100-500)	Large (Over 500)	Total
20	Food and kindred products	138 (36.7)	516 (74.6)	296 (88.2)	950 (67.7)
21	Tobacco products	346 (7.7)	7 (65.1)	34 (51.6)	41 (50.9)
22	Textile mill products	13 (13.8)	37 (38.0)	36 (84.4)	86 (37.0)
23	Apparel and other textile products	9 (1.9)	10 (2.5)	38 (100.0)	57 (6.2)
24	Lumber and wood products	23 (27.1)	26 (52.3)	22 (81.6)	71 (44.0)
25	Furniture and fixtures	7 (6.7)	55 (42.9)	49 (91.0)	112 (37.8)
26	Paper and allied products	46 (36.1)	209 (79.0)	179 (100.0)	434 (76.0)
27	Printing and publishing	18 (5.1)	87 (27.9)	437 (75.6)	542 (43.7)
28	Chemicals and allied products	101 (51.9)	153 (79.8)	553 (95.4)	807 (83.5)
29	Petroleum and coal products	9 (43.4)	52 (97.7)	122 (100.0)	183 (93.5)
30	Rubber and miscellaneous plastics	24 (17.3)	115 (60.0)	186 (91.0)	325 (60.8)
31	Leather and leather products	2 (5.0)	14 (15.8)	10 (39.2)	26 (17.0)
32	Stone, clay and glass products	47 (26.0)	256 (83.7)	205 (96.1)	508 (72.6)
33	Primary metals	53 (43.3)	198 (89.4)	995 (99.0)	1,246 (92.4)
34	Fabricated metals	135 (30.2)	393 (76.2)	385 (100.0)	914 (67.7)
35	Machinery, except electrical	62 (22.8)	272 (73.5)	878 (97.7)	1,212 (78.7)
36	Electric and electronic equipment	24 (24.0)	135 (40.8)	1,010 (94.4)	1,169 (77.9)
37	Transportation equipment	18 (23.7)	100 (68.5)	993 (99.3)	1,112 (90.8)
38	Instruments	21 (24.6)	32 (45.1)	223 (98.4)	277 (71.8)
39	Miscellaneous manufacturing	25 (18.3)	42 (27.8)	53 (56.9)	121 (31.4)

SOURCE: NIOSH Occupational Hazards Survey, 1977.

Table 50: Number and Percent of Plants and Employees in Plants Covered by Periodic Medical Examinations

SIC Code	Industry	Small (8-99)	Plants Medium (100-500)	Large (Over 500)	Total
20	Food and kindred products	2,497 (19.5)	1,381 (46.3)	300 (74.3)	4,178 (25.8)
21	Tobacco products		16 (47.1)	25 (62.5)	41 (20.9)
22	Textile mill products	232 (8.6)	120 (24.2)	18 (48.6)	370 (11.5)
23	Apparel and other textile products	507 (3.8)	294 (12.6)	14 (31.8)	815 (5.2)
24	Lumber and wood products	267 (9.6)	44 (15.8)	13 (37.1)	325 (10.5)
25	Furniture and fixtures	91 (2.4)	88 (12.9)	43 (56.6)	222 (4.8)
26	Paper and allied products	268 (8.3)	585 (41.6)	62 (30.1)	915 (18.8)
27	Printing and publishing	104 (0.9)	260 (17.4)	198 (537)	562 (4.1)
28	Chemicals and allied products	1,314 (24.5)	342 (37.1)	275 (58.9)	1,931 (28.6)
29	Petroleum and coal products	89 (12.8)	130 (55.3)	56 (88.9)	276 (27.8)
30	Rubber and miscellaneous plastics	1,342 (29.7)	172 (17.6)	65 (43.9)	1,579 (28.0)
31	Leather and leather products	62 (5.3)	32 (7.3)	3 (8.8)	96 (5.8)
32	Stone, clay and glass products	1,619 (25.4)	455 (31.7)	31 (21.7)	2,106 (26.5)
33	Primary metals	417 (11.1)	431 (46.7)	299 (82.4)	1,147 (22.8)
34	Fabricated metals	1,910 (11.5)	809 (30.6)	22 (56.7)	2,949 (15.0)
35	Machinery, except electrical	605 (5.1)	543 (29.3)	383 (66.3)	1,532 (10.8)
36	Electric and electronic equipment	272 (8.8)	262 (17.3)	254 (54.9)	788 (15.5)
37	Transportation equipment	215 (8.7)	96 (15.5)	277 (74.7)	588 (17.0)
38	Instruments	168 (5.2)	98 (26.8)	89 (45.2)	355 (9.3)
39	Miscellaneous manufacturing	156 (3.1)	93 (12.8)	50 (52.6)	299 (5.2)

Table 50: continued

SIC Code	Industry	Small (8-99)	Employees in Plants (thousands) Medium (100-500)	Large (Over 500)	Total
20	Food and kindred products	102 (27.2)	321 (46.4)	228 (68.3)	653 (46.5)
21	Tobacco products	—	5 (50.4)	55 (83.7)	60 (74.7)
22	Textile mill products	7 (8.4)	32 (33.4)	12 (28.4)	52 (22.6)
23	Apparel and other textile products	25 (5.0)	56 (14.9)	19 (50.0)	100 (10.9)
24	Lumber and wood products	8 (9.6)	8 (15.1)	12 (44.7)	28 (17.1)
25	Furniture and fixtures	5 (4.4)	22 (16.8)	32 (60.4)	59 (20.0)
26	Paper and allied products	15 (12.0)	118 (44.5)	80 (44.9)	213 (37.4)
27	Printing and publishing	9 (2.7)	82 (26.1)	320 (55.5)	411 (33.2)
28	Chemicals and allied products	56 (28.9)	73 (38.0)	391 (67.6)	520 (53.9)
29	Petroleum and coal products	4 (22.4)	35 (64.8)	118 (96.8)	157 (80.4)
30	Rubber and miscellaneous plastics	22 (16.1)	47 (24.3)	132 (64.5)	201 (37.6)
31	Leather and leather products	1 (2.7)	5 (6.0)	6 (25.1)	13 (8.3)
32	Stone, clay and glass products	48 (26.5)	122 (39.9)	124 (58.2)	294 (42.0)
33	Primary metals	16 (13.2)	113 (51.1)	952 (94.8)	1,081 (80.2)
34	Fabricated metals	77 (17.2)	192 (37.3)	235 (61.0)	505 (37.4)
35	Machinery, except electrical	23 (8.6)	118 (31.9)	741 (82.4)	883 (57.3)
36	Electric and electronic equipment	11 (10.8)	56 (17.1)	874 (81.6)	941 (62.7)
37	Transportation equipment	9 (12.2)	25 (17.2)	880 (88.0)	914 (74.7)
38	Instruments	5 (5.5)	22 (30.8)	116 (51.0)	143 (37.0)
39	Miscellaneous manufacturing	3 (2.4)	21 (13.9)	54 (56.9)	77 (20.2)

SOURCE: NIOSH Occupational Hazards Survey, 1977.

Food, Beverages, and Tobacco Industries. Workers in the food, beverages, and tobacco industries are exposed to a variety of biological and industrial hazards. However, these industries have not been major targets of OSHA regulations in the past. In spite of that, the industry has provided better than average health care for its employees, as can be seen from the results of the NIOSH survey.[42]

Statistics regarding the size of these industries are presented in Tables 43-50.

Eight companies within these industries responded to the F&S survey. Plant size varied from 450 to 4000 employees and the plants were located throughout the United States. Five of the respondents were physicians and three, registered nurses. The majority of the physicians and the nurses were full-time employees. Seven out of the eight companies had full-time medical departments.

The screening regimens reported are summarized in Table 51. Respondents estimated screening costs between $28.00 and $100.00 per employee per year. Average annual costs were $69.50 per employee.

Tests considered by the respondents as valuable in this area include: urinalysis (25 percent), pulmonary function, blood analysis, vision screening, and audiometry.

The Textile Industry. The textile industry has been the target of several OSHA campaigns to protect workers' health from such problems as excessive noise and byssinosis (brown lung disease) caused by cotton dust. Current cotton dust standards, as proposed by OSHA, are expected to cost the industry nearly $1 billion and the noise abatement problem perhaps even more.

The textile industry's profit margins are about 3 cents on the dollar, which is nearly half of the average of manufacturing in general. Investments made to meet health and safety standards, are strongly opposed by the industry, since it believes that it would be difficult to pass along the costs to the consumer in view of cheaper imports.

The textile industry is located primarily in the South and it employs approximately 765,300 production workers. Also, it is estimated that there are 232,000 retired employees. The majority of the textile mills employ fewer than 100 workers. There are about 2175 facilities with more than 100 workers and only 1093 facilities with more than 250 workers.

Approximately 600,000 of textile workers are exposed to cotton dust. Also, the majority of these workers are exposed to detrimental noise levels. The medical surveillance program adopted by the textile industry should therefore include, in addition to a physical examination and medical history, pulmonary function testing and audiometry. The degree of availability of such tests in this industry is shown in Tables 22, 24, 25, 28, 38, and 41, as estimated by the NIOSH survey.[42] The F&S survey includes six responses from the textile industry representing 132,000 workers. Five of the respondents were industrial physicians and one was a director of nursing. Plant size varied from 2000 to 60,000 employees; all had a full-time medical department and five such departments were headed by a full-time physician. A summary of the screening regimen is shown in Table 52.

Table 51: Testing Regimen as Reported by Respondents in the Food and Tobacco Industry

	Percent	General Employees	Employees in Hazardous Jobs
Testing Frequency			
Preemployment only		62.5%	25%
Preemployment and annual			12.5
Annual		12.5	50
Other (implies more often or for different groups)		25	12.5
Type of Tests			
Medical history	100		
Physical examination	87.5		
X-ray	25		
Pulmonary function	25		
Clinical laboratory	87.5		
Blood	87.5		
Urine	87.5		
Sputum	12.5		
Audiometry	50		
Vision tests	37.5		
EKG	37.5		
Performer of Screening			
In-house medical department	62.5		
Single outside service company	12.5		
Multiple outside providers	12.5		
All of the above	25.0		
Future Performer of Screening			
In-house resources	62.5		
Outside providers	37.5		
Special Equipment in Place			
PFT	25		
Audiometer	25		
X-ray	25		
Vision	25		
EKG	37.5		

SOURCE: F&S Survey.

Table 52: Testing Regimen as Reported by Respondents in the Textile Industry

	Percent	General Employees	Employees in Hazardous Jobs
Testing Frequency			
Preemployment only		66.6%	—
Preemployment and annual		16.7	16.7%
Annual			50
Biannual			33.3
Other (implies more often or for different groups)		33.3	50
Type of Tests			
Medical history	100		
Physical examination	50		
X-ray	16.7		
Pulmonary function	100		
Clinical laboratory	66.7		
Blood	33.3		
Urine	66.7	(One respondent used urine tests in special situations only)	
Sputum	—		
Audiometry	100		
Vision tests	33.3		
Performer of Screening			
In-house medical department	83.3		
Single outside service company			
Multiple outside providers			
All of the above	16.7		
Future Performer of Screening			
In-house resources	100		
Outside providers			
Special Equipment in Place			
PFT	83.3		
Audiometer	83.3		
Routine laboratory	50		
X-ray	16.7		
Vision	16.7		

SOURCE: F&S Survey.

All the respondents to the survey represented large plants and their programs should not be considered as the norm for the industry. The NIOSH survey that reports data for the 1972-1974 period estimates that only 3.6 percent of all textile mills and 21.6 percent of those employing more than 500 persons incorporate pulmonary function in their screening regimen, and 7.3 and 21.6 percent, respectively, incorporate audiometric evaluations. All the facilities from the F&S survey included pulmonary function and audiometry in their testing regimen, as can be seen in Table 52. Interestingly, nearly all facilities own some special screening devices, such as pulmonary function testing equipment and audiometers.

The screening costs reported range from $15 to $100 per employee annually. The majority of the respondents perform employee screening in-house and plan to do so in the future.

As expected, the most common tests were those for pulmonary function and hearing. However, textile workers are also exposed to many other chemical hazards, such as heavy metals and their compounds, ketones, and isocyanates. Therefore a more complete testing regimen is also desirable. The majority of the survey respondents also included urinalysis as part of their screening regimen. The respondents recommended several additional tests, such as EKG, SMA-12, vision tests, and sputum cytology.

Finally, all of the respondents were from North and South Carolina, which is no surprise, since the industry is now concentrated in this region.

Paper and Wood Products Industries. Workers in the paper industry are exposed to various hazardous agents, such as ozone, sulfur dioxide, sulfuric acid, and zinc chloride. Statistics regarding the size of these industries are given in Tables 42-45.

F&S received 12 replies from health professionals in these industries, representing more than 131,300 employees and including plants with 500 workers and companies with 50,000 workers. Replies came from physicians and nurses in equal proportions. All but two of the respondents stated that their companies or plants had a formally established unit.

Testing regimens and equipment in place are shown in Table 53.

The respondents to the F&S survey indicated that special tests are performed by more facilities than estimated by the NIOSH survey. Also in the majority of the companies tests were performed by an in-house medical department that appeared to be well equipped. Respondents also indicated that they plan to use in-house resources in the future.

Costs of the screening program per employee per annum ranged from $20 to $250, with an average cost of $68. The respondents expressed the intention to acquire such equipment as pulmonary function equipment (25 percent), tonometers, audiometers, and physiotherapy equipment. They recommended that the following tests be performed in their industries: pulmonary function (68.8 percent), audiometry (58.3 percent), chest x-rays (58.3 percent), blood evaluations (50 percent), vision screening (41.7 percent), EKG (25 percent), and other clinical evaluations (33.3 percent).

Table 53: Testing Regimen as Reported by Respondents in the Paper and Wood Products Industries

	Percent	General Employees	Employees in Hazardous Jobs
Testing Frequency			
Preemployment only		50%	25%
Preemployment and annual		25	25
Annual		16.7	33.3
Biannual		—	8.3
Other (at terminations)		16.7	25
Type of Tests			
Medical history	100		
Physical examination	91.7		
X-ray	66.7		
Pulmonary function	50		
Clinical laboratory	83.3		
Blood	50		
Urine	83.3		
Sputum	—		
Audiometry	83.3		
Vision tests	63.6		
EKG	41.6		
Performer of Screening			
In-house medical department	63.6		
Single outside service company	8.3		
Multiple outside providers	8.3		
All of the above	25		
Future Performer of Screening			
In-house resources	66.7		
Outside providers	25.0		
Special Equipment in Place			
Routine laboratory	33.3		
Audiometer	83.3		
Vision	41.6		
PFT	66.7		
EKG	41.6		

SOURCE: F&S Survey.

Chemicals and Allied Products. Workers in the chemical industry are exposed to myriads of substances, many extremely hazardous. As a result, workplace conditions in this industry have been scrutinized by a number of regulatory agencies for some time. Statistics regarding the size of this industry are presented in Tables 43-50.

As expected, the majority of the replies to the F&S survey within the manufacturing industries category came from the chemicals industry. The contributions of the 59 respondents are summarized in Table 54. Plant and company size represented by the respondents varied from 98 to 82,000 workers. All in all, 570,960 workers were represented. The majority of the respondents were physicians (67.8 percent) and 65 percent of them were full-time company employees. Also, 14.7 percent of the respondents were nurses, with 87.5 percent being full-time employees. Approximately 14.7 percent of the respondents were industrial hygienists and 50 percent of them were full-time employees. Nearly all plants (96.6 percent) participating in the F&S survey had a full-time medical department.

As we can see from Table 54 the majority of the plants provide annual examinations for their employees. Also those who provide the tests use a fairly comprehensive screening regimen. The majority of the plants performed the tests in-house and about 50 percent of them had a well-equipped medical department.

Compared to the estimates of the NIOSH survey (see Table 55), the F&S results show a significant increase in the number of large plants performing certain types of specialized tests, such as x-ray (98.3 versus 45 percent), pulmonary function (72.8 versus 25.3 percent), vision screening (62.7 versus 45 percent), and blood (100 versus 35.1 percent) and urine (93.2 versus 24.4 percent) tests.

Quoted annual costs per employee ranged from $15 to $225, with the average being $95.40.

Equipment that the respondents considered incorporating in their departments included: computers (15.3 percent), pulmonary function devices (13.6 percent), and EKGs and stress testing systems (13.6 percent). Other tests mentioned include: sputum cytology, urinalysis, drug monitoring, vision screening, chest x-ray, toxic agents screen, carcinogenic screen, biochemical screen, audiometry, semen analysis, and electromyography.

Screening procedures considered valuable by the respondents in their field of practice include: pulmonary function screening (16.9 percent), x-ray (15.3 percent), blood tests (13.6 percent), audiometry (11.7 percent), urinalysis (10.2 percent), EKG (10.2 percent), and vision screening (6.8 percent).

A large subset of the chemical industry is the pharmaceutical industry in which employees are exposed to numerous natural and synthetic agents that are potential toxins. Some studies suggest that there may be an increased incidence of cancer among pharmaceutical production workers.

Table 54: Testing Regimen as Reported by Respondents in the Chemicals Industry

	Percent	General Employees	Employees in Hazardous Jobs
Testing Frequency			
Preemployment only		30.5%	14.3%
Preemployment and annual		0	0
Annual		54	67.8
Biannual		23.7	18.6
Other		28.8	20.3
Type of Tests			
Medical History	100.0		
Physical examination	89.8		
X-ray	98.3		
Pulmonary function	72.8		
Clinical laboratory	100.0		
Blood	100.0		
Urine	93.2		
Sputum	10.2		
Stool	8.5		
Pap smear	8.5		
Audiometry	62.7		
Vision tests	62.7		
Tonometry	18.6		
EKG	62.7		
Proctosigmoidoscopy	10.2		
Other (urine cytology, liver function)	33.9		
Performer of Screening			
In-house medical department	84.7		
Single outside service company	15.2		
Multiple outside providers	15.2		
All of the above	5.0		
Future Performer of Screening			
In-house resources	84.7		
Outside providers	27.1		
Special Equipment in Place			
Audiometer	55.9		
EKG	50.8		
Vision testing	50.8		
Spirometer	49.1		
X-ray	33.9		
Chemical laboratory	18.6		
Blood	13.5		
Urine	10.2		

SOURCE: F&S Survey.

Table 55: Summary of Number and Percent of Plants and Employees in Plants Covered by Special Medical Services—Chemicals Industry

	Chemicals Industry				Employees (thousands)			
	Small (8–99)	Medium (100–500)	Large (Over 500)	Total	Small (8–99)	Medium (100–500)	Large (Over 500)	Total
Formally established health unit	210 (3.9)	391 (42.4)	371 (79.4)	972 (14.4)	13 (6.9)	100 (52.2)	526 (90.8)	639 (66.1)
Regularly record health information about new employees	4,015 (75)	923 (100)	467 (100)	5,405 (80.2)	147 (75)	191 (100)	579 (100)	917 (94.9)
Require preplacement physical examinations	2,252 (42.1)	661 (77.6)	416 (89.1)	3,329 (49.4)	101 (51.9)	153 (79.8)	553 (95.4)	807 (83.5)
Provide periodic medical examinations	1,314 (24.5)	342 (37.1)	275 (58.9)	1,931 (28.6)	56 (28.9)	73 (38)	391 (67.6)	320 (53.9)
Provide audiometric examinations	516 (9.6)	189 (20.5)	225 (54.6)	959 (14.2)	22 (11)	48 (25.4)	379 (65.5)	449 (46.5)
Provide periodic pulmonary function screening	600 (11.2)	64 (6.9)	118 (25.3)	781 (11.6)	25 (12.6)	20 (10.2)	292 (50.5)	337 (34.9)
Provide ophthalmological examinations	450 (8.4)	204 (22.1)	210 (45)	864 (12.8)	19 (9.6)	45 (23.5)	352 (60.9)	416 (43.1)
Provide x-ray examinations	840 (15.7)	234 (25.4)	210 (45)	1,284 (19)	38 (19.5)	57 (30)	352 (60.9)	448 (46.4)
Provide periodic urine tests	800 (14.9)	139 (15.1)	114 (24.4)	1,054 (15.6)	26 (13.1)	31 (16.2)	282 (48.9)	340 (35.2)
Provide periodic blood tests	914 (17.1)	118 (12.8)	164 (35.1)	1,197 (17.8)	34 (17.6)	25 (13)	314 (54.2)	373 (38.7)

Petroleum and Coal Products. Petroleum workers are exposed to numerous workplace hazards, such as benzene, toluene, heavy metals and their compounds, sulfur dioxide, and fluorides. Many of these substances are systemic toxins and suspected carcinogens.

The petroleum and coal products industry employs 144,400 workers (100,200 of them involved in production). There are 720 establishments within this industry and about 37 percent of them employ more than 100 workers (see Tables 43-50).

The NIOSH survey[42] estimated that 27.8 percent of all plants in the petroleum and coal industries provided medical examinations to their employees. Nearly 89 percent of the plants employing more than 500 workers reported providing such examinations and 100 percent of such plants are estimated to have a formally established health unit.

Eleven companies in this industry replied to the F&S survey, representing 63,100 employees. Seven of the respondents were physicians, six of whom were full-time employees. Nine of the companies had full-time medical departments. Respondents represented various plant sizes from 500 workers to large company headquarters overseeing thousands. Testing regimens and procedures and providers employed are summarized in Table 56.

All respondents reported providing some type of periodic health screening service to their employees. Nearly all reported taking a medical history and providing a physical examination during a medical screening procedure. Also, all reported providing clinical laboratory tests, such as blood and urine examinations. About 36.4 percent reported performing sputum examinations, a high rate compared to other industries. This is not surprising, since petroleum workers have been found to have a higher risk of lung cancer.

These results, compared with the finding of the NIOSH survey,[42] are not surprising. The only discrepancies arise in the adoption of audiometric and ophthalmologic examinations (our sample indicates lesser adoption of such tests) and in the popularity of blood and urine tests (our sample indicates a higher level of adoption of such tests).

Unfortunately, not enough of the respondents quoted annual costs per employee to calculate average values.

Table 56: Testing Regimen as Reported by Respondents in the Petroleum and Coal Industry

	Percent	General Employees	Employees in Hazardous Jobs
Testing Frequency			
Preemployment only		45.4%	9%
Preemployment and annual		18.2	36.4
Annual		9.0	27.3
Biannual			9.0
Other		54.5	45.4
Type of Tests			
Medical history	90.9		
Physical examination	90.9		
X-ray	72.7		
Pulmonary function	72.7		
Clinical laboratory	100.0		
Blood	100.0		
Urine	90.9		
Sputum	36.4		
Audiometry	45.4		
Vision tests	36.4		
Other (EKG, Stool, SMA-24, SMA-20, Pap smear, SMA-12)	36.4		
Performer of Screening			
In-house medical department	45.4		
Single outside service company	27.3		
Multiple outside providers	18.2		
All of the above	18.2		
Future Performer of Screening			
In-house resources	45.4		
Outside providers	45.4		
Special Equipment in Place			
X-ray	54.5		
EKG	54.5		
PFT	72.7		
Routine laboratory	45.4		
SMAC-20	9.0		
Lead testing	9.0		
Audiometer	63.6		
Vision	36.4		

SOURCE: F&S Survey

Primary Metals Industry. Employees in the primary metals industry are exposed to various hazardous substances, such as coke oven emissions, coal tars, metals (such as beryllium, brass, lead, magnesium, nickel, thallium, tin, and zinc) and their compounds, including arsenic. Statistics regarding the size of this industry are given in Tables 43-50.

There were 35 respondents to the F&S survey from this industry. Respondents represented a range of plant and company sizes from 203 to 12,000 employees, with the total number of workers being 121,553. The majority of the respondents (80 percent) were physicians, 42.8 percent of whom were full-time company employees. Of the remaining respondents, 14.3 percent were nurses (80 percent of them were full-time employees) and the rest were full-time employed industrial hygienists. Nearly all of the plants (94.3 percent) had a full-time medical department.

Screening regimens and the type and frequency of specialized tests performed by the respondents are given in Table 57. Quoted annual costs per employee ranged from $5 to $300, with an average cost of $81.70.

Nearly 28.6 percent of the respondents said they were reviewing computerized screening equipment and automated recording and storage systems with the intent to incorporate them into their practice.

Tests deemed valuable to the practice of the respondents to the F&S survey include: audiometry (31.4 percent), chest x-rays (25.7 percent), pulmonary function screening (22.9 percent), and vision screening (22.9 percent).

Compared to the NIOSH survey[42] estimates as shown in various tables in chapters 8 and 9, the F&S survey indicates a significant increase in the performance of such tests as: pulmonary function (60 versus 38 percent), x-ray (94.3 versus 78.4 percent), blood tests (74.3 versus 43.3 percent), and urinalysis (88.6 versus 51 percent). On the other hand, audiometry and vision screening was performed by fewer plants in the F&S survey than the NIOSH estimate (see Tables 25 and 31).

Fabricated Metals Industry. Employees in this industry are exposed to metal fumes, solvents, acid or alkaline substances, heavy metals, and cutting oils. The industry is dominated by small firms of less than 100 employees who employ 27.4 percent of the work force within this industry. More detailed statistics regarding this industry can be found in Tables 43-50.

There were 10 replies to the F&S survey from the fabricated metals industry. The total number of employees represented was 25,330. The size of plants varied from 260 to 9000 employees. Approximately 40 percent of the respondents were physicians (75 percent were full-time employees) and 60 percent were nurses, all of whom were full-time employees. Also, 90 percent of the plants had a full-time medical department.

Screening regimens used by the respondents and the type and frequency of tests incorporated in such regimens are given in Table 58.

Quoted annual costs per employee ranged from $25 to $150, with an average cost of $75.

Table 57: Testing Regimen as Reported by Respondents in the Primary Metals Industry

	Percent	General Employees	Employees in Hazardous Jobs
Testing Frequency			
Preemployment only		31.4%	14.3%
Preemployment and annual		11.4	5.7
Annual		48.6	62.8
Biannual		25.7	45.7
Other		25.7	22.8
Type of Tests			
Medical history	97.1		
Physical examination	97.1		
X-ray	94.3		
Pulmonary function	60.0		
Clinical laboratory	88.6		
Blood	74.3		
Urine	88.6		
Sputum	34.3		
Audiometry	60.0		
Vision tests	48.6		
EKG	31.4		
Other	31.4		
Performer of Screening			
In-house medical department	94.3		
Single outside service company	17.1		
Multiple outside providers	20.0		
All of the above	5.7		
Future Performer of Screening			
In-house resources	82.8		
Outside providers	17.1		
Special Equipment in Place			
Spirometers	70.2		
X-ray	57.1		
Audiometers	48.6		
Vision testing	48.6		
EKG	31.4		
Urine testing	20.0		
Blood testing	11.4		

SOURCE: F&S Survey.

Table 58: Testing Regimen as Reported by Respondents in the Fabricated Metals Industry

	Percent	General Employees	Employees in Hazardous Jobs
Testing Frequency			
Preemployment only		50%	1%
Preemployment and annual		1	0
Annual		30	60
Biannual		30	20
Other		30	30
Type of Tests			
Medical history	90		
Physical examination	90		
X-ray	50		
Pulmonary function	50		
Clinical laboratory	100		
Blood	70		
Urine	100		
EKG	50		
Audiometry	70		
Vision tests	60		
Other (serology-VDRL, lead, (stool, procto, pap)	30		
Performer of Screening			
In-house medical department	100		
Single outside service company	20		
Multiple outside providers	30		
All of the above	0		
Future Performer of Screening			
In-house resources	90		
Outside providers	30		
Special Equipment in Place			
Audiometers	50		
Vision tests	50		
X-ray	50		
EKG	50		
Spirometers	40		

SOURCE: F&S Survey.

Machinery, Except Electrical. Statistics regarding the size of this industry are presented in Tables 43-50.

There were 24 survey replies in this category. Respondents represented small plants and large corporations employing from 325 to 44,000 people. The total number of workers employed by the companies of the respondents was 88,244. Nearly 87.5 percent of the respondents said that their company had a full-time medical department. Approximately 37.5 percent of the respondents were industrial physicians and 44 percent of these were employed full time and 56 percent, part time. Nurses represented 58.3 percent of the respondents and 71.4 percent were employed full time and 38.6 percent were part-time employees.

The frequency and type of tests performed are given in Table 59. This table also shows the type of equipment available at the plant facility. In addition 8.3 percent of the respondents said that other equipment, such as vision testers, audiometers, EKGs, and blood testing devices, would be desirable and one respondent is interested in a computerized record keeping system.

Tests deemed helpful to health professionals in this area include: audiometry (41.7 percent), spirometry (37.5 percent), vision screening (29.2 percent), blood pressure measurement (25 percent), blood analysis (20.8 percent), EKG (12.5 percent), and urinalysis (12.5 percent).

Annual costs per employee were quoted at a high of $200 to a low of $25, with the average being $62.00.

Electrical and Electronic. Workers in this industry are exposed to lead and its compounds, mercury and its compounds, beryllium, platinum, selenium, and graphite. Statistics regarding the size of this industry are given in Tables 43-50.

There were 39 respondents to the F&S survey from this industry and five of them were manufacturers of batteries. Plant and company sizes varied from 180 to 180,000 employees. The total number of employees represented were 376,830. Nearly 59 percent of the respondents were physicians, 56.5 percent of whom were full-time employees of the company. The remainder of the respondents (41 percent) were nursing personnel and 89.7 percent of them were full-time employees. Also 89.7 percent of the companies had a full-time medical department.

The types of tests performed during a routine medical screening procedure and the frequency of such tests, as reported by the respondents, are given in Table 60. The same table lists all specialized medical equipment listed by the respondent as available in the plant's medical department. Equipment considered for addition to existing facilities included: computers (7.7 percent), devices to measure stamina and agility (7.9 percent), exercise rooms and whirlpool bath, computerized EKG, x-ray system.

Table 59: Testing Regimen as Reported by Respondents in the Machinery, Except Electrical, Industry

	Percent	General Employees	Employees in Hazardous Jobs
Testing Frequency			
Preemployment only		62.5%	12.5%
Preemployment and annual		12.5	12.5
Annual		12.5	45.8
Biannual		12.5	4.2
Other		16.7	20.8
Type of Tests			
Medical history	83.3		
Physical examination	83.3		
X-ray	54.7		
Pulmonary function	29.2		
Clinical laboratory	75.0		
Blood	41.7		
Urine	75.0		
EKG	16.7		
Audiometry	62.5		
Vision tests	50.0		
Performer of Screening			
In-house medical department	75.0		
Single outside service company	20.8		
Multiple outside providers	37.5		
Future Performer of Screening			
In-house resources	79.2		
Outside providers	25.0		
Equipment in Situ			
Audiometer	62.5		
Vision tests	50.0		
Spirometer	29.2		
X-ray	16.7		
EKG	16.7		
Blood pressure	12.5		
Clinical laboratory	12.5		

SOURCE: F&S Survey.

Table 60: Testing Regimen as Reported by Respondents in the Electrical and Electronic Industry

	Percent	General Employees	Employees in Hazardous Jobs
Testing Frequency			
Preemployment only		71.8%	25.6%
Preemployment and annual		5.1	5.1
Annual		15.4	15.4
Biannual		10.2	20.5
Other		23.0	23.0
Type of Tests			
Medical history	97.4		
Physical examination	92.3		
X-ray	51.3		
Pulmonary function	25.6		
Clinical laboratory	94.9		
Blood	64.1		
Urine	94.9		
EKG	17.9		
Audiometry	30.7		
Vision tests	17.9		
Other (sputum, serology, SMA-12, immunization)	23.0		
Performer of Screening			
In-house medical department	79.5		
Single outside service company	25.6		
Multiple outside providers	17.9		
All of the above	7.7		
Future Performer of Screening			
In-house resources	69.2		
Outside providers	25.6		
Equipment in Situ			
EKG	50.0		
Vision	41.0		
Audiometer	38.4		
X-ray	35.9		
Spirometer	35.9		
Clinical laboratory	10.2		
Blood test	7.7		
Urine test	7.7		

SOURCE: F&S Survey.

The respondents also listed several medical procedures considered most applicable within their industry. Techniques mentioned include: chest x-ray (17.9 percent), pulmonary function screening (17.9 percent), blood tests (15.3 percent), audiometry (12.8 percent), urinalysis (12.8 percent), EKG (12.8 percent), vision tests (10.2 percent), SMA-12 (7.7 percent), heavy metal screening (7.7 percent), SMA-20, SMAC, sputum cytology.

Quotes for screening costs per annum per employee ranged from a low of $2.00 to a high of $160.00, with the average cost being $48.40.

Transportation Equipment Manufacturers Industry. Transportation equipment manufacturers include: automotive, shipbuilding, and aircraft and space vehicles manufacture.

High incidence of lung cancer has been associated with shipbuilding, probably because the workers were exposed to asbestos. Most cases appear 20 years after employment terminated, which indicates the ability of carcinogens to induce disease after long periods of time.

Standards and controls introduced in this area since World War II are cited as having solved the problem, but epidemiological studies have not shown this to be the case. It has been theorized that other carcinogens, in addition to asbestos, existing in the shipbuilding area are also responsible for the increased rates of lung cancer and other cancers, such as those of the larynx, the oropharynx, and upper gastrointestinal tract.

There were 39 respondents representing this industry. Plant and company size varied from 20 to 880,000 employees. The total number of employees represented was 1,155,458. Nearly 77 percent of all respondents were physicians and 73.3 percent of them were full-time employees. The remainder were industrial hygienists (5.1 percent) and nursing personnel (15.4 percent). Nearly 67 percent of the nurses and 50 percent of the hygienists were full-time employees.

The type of tests performed during a periodic screening procedure and the frequency of health screening are given in Table 61. Equipment available at the company medical department are also listed in Table 61.

Quoted screening costs per employee per annum varied from $15 to $260, with the average cost being $84.80.

The respondents listed several devices as potentially useful in their practice, such as x-ray systems (12.8 percent), computers (10.2 percent), spirometers (7.7 percent), and audiometers, tonometers, clinical laboratory instruments, whirlpools, and treadmills. Equipment deemed relevant to the screening programs for this particular industry included: audiometers (30.8 percent), blood tests (20.5 percent), vision testers (17.9 percent), x-ray equipment (15.4 percent), spirometers (15.4 percent), EKG (10.2 percent), and urinalysis systems and SMA-24.

Table 61: Testing Regimen as Reported by Respondents in the Transportation Equipment Manufacturers Industry

	Percent	General Employees	Employees in Hazardous Jobs
Testing Frequency			
Preemployment only		56.4%	7.7%
Preemployment and annual		17.9	5.1
Annual		20.5	56.4
Biannual		2.6	15.4
Other		30.8	23.0
Type of Tests			
Medical history	97.4		
Physical examination	84.6		
X-ray	87.2		
Pulmonary function	30.7		
Clinical laboratory	84.6		
Blood	84.6		
Urine	51.2		
Sputum	5.1		
Audiometry	41.0		
Vision tests	35.9		
EKG	23.0		
Other (treadmill, hand grip, etc.)	25.6		
Performer of Screening			
In-house medical department	82.0		
Single outside service company	18.0		
Multiple outside providers	20.5		
All of the above	5.1		
Future Performer of Screening			
In-house resources	82.0		
Outside providers	15.4		
Equipment in Situ			
X-ray	53.8		
Audiometer	48.7		
Pulmonary function	48.7		
Vision	46.1		
EKG	43.6		
Blood	7.7		
Urine	7.7		

SOURCE: F&S Survey.

Services

Medical surveillance efforts in the services sector are usually age-related, voluntary screening programs, often made available to special employees, such as executives, and mostly consisting of evaluations of the cardiovascular system and screening for such disorders as diabetes, hypertension, and pulmonary diseases.

However, nonmanufacturing workers are also faced with the risk of having their health jeopardized by occupational hazards. One inadvertent hazard, the result of energy conservation efforts, has been created from indoor air pollution in heat-sealed homes and offices. In the past this type of pollution was not considered a serious health hazard because buildings were continuously ventilated because of poor insulation. But recent advances in building materials and techniques has reduced outside air infiltration to minimal levels and ventilation has been also curtailed in an effort to conserve energy.

The lack of ventilation results in build-up of dangerous levels of pollutants emitted by building materials and home furnishings. Radon, a radioactive gas given off from rock, water, soil, and certain building materials, has been found in homes and offices in concentrations above those considered occupationally safe. Other harmful substances, such as formaldehyde and asbestos, are given off by carpeting, drapes, and building materials. Also gas stoves and other appliances emit harmful air pollutants, such as carbon monoxide and nitrogen dioxide, which can become a serious health hazard if not properly vented. Other products, such as sprays, cleaning agents, solvents, adhesives, paint and smoke, continuously pollute the indoor air.

Special populations within the services sector also find themselves in hazardous environments, particularly hospital and laboratory workers. In this subsection three service industries, public utilities, insurance and finance, and hospitals, are discussed in some detail.

Utilities. There were 39 respondents to the F&S survey from this industry. Plant and company size varied from 200 to 104,000 employees with a total of 326,900 employees. Nearly 82 percent of the respondents were physicians and 50 percent of them were full-time company employees. About 7.7 percent of the respondents were nurses employed on a full-time basis. Also, 82 percent of the companies and plants in this group had a full-time medical department.

The type of medical screening regimen adopted by this industry is given in Table 62. This table also lists the medical equipment incorporated in the various medical facilities.

Quoted screening costs per employee per year varied from $7.50 to $300, with an average of $61.80.

The results of the F&S survey are in line with the data produced by the NIOSH survey.[42] Both sources indicate that this industry, although it has few employees who are exposed to hazardous materials, have an active employee health surveillance program (see Tables 62 and 63).

Table 62: Testing Regimen as Reported by Respondents in the Utilities Industry

	Percent	General Employees	Employees in Hazardous Jobs
Testing Frequency			
Preemployment only		48.7%	30.7%
Preemployment and annual		12.8	5.1
Annual		10.2	35.9
Biannual		15.4	10.2
Other		25.6	35.9
Type of Tests			
Medical history	94.9		
Physical examination	82.0		
X-ray	60.0		
Pulmonary function	25.6		
Clinical laboratory	82.0		
Blood	48.7		
Urine	82.0		
Sputum	5.1		
Audiometry	28.2		
Vision tests	41.0		
EKG	17.9		
Other	15.4		
Performer of Screening			
In-house medical department	79.5		
Single outside service company	23.0		
Multiple outside providers	43.5		
All of the above	12.8		
Future Performer of Screening			
In-house resources	53.8		
Outside providers	30.7		
Equipment in Situ			
Audiometry	53.8		
EKG	51.3		
PFT	41.0		
Vision	38.5		
Laboratory	25.6		
Blood	7.7		
Urine	5.1		
X-ray	20.5		
Sigmoidoscope	7.7		

SOURCE: F&S Survey

Covered by Special Medical Services—Utilities

	Public Utility Plants				Employees (thousands)			
	Small (8-99)	Medium (100-500)	Large (Over 500)	Total	Small (8-99)	Medium (100-500)	Large (Over 500)	Total
Formally established health unit	439 (0.4)	430 (4.3)	423 (59.9)	1,292 (1.1)	17.2 (0.7)	71.6 (4.1)	1,200.7 (78.5)	1,289.6 (22.4)
Regularly record health information about new employees	22,709 (20.2)	4,942 (49.6)	706 (100)	28,357 (23.1)	688.1 (27.5)	897.2 (51.8)	1,530.0 (100)	3,115.4 (54)
Require preplacement physical examinations	17,558 (15.6)	4,339 (43.5)	657 (93.1)	22,554 (18.3)	537.5 (21.5)	773.3 (44.6)	1,390.1 (90.9)	2,700.9 (46.8)
Provide periodic medical examinations	11,517 (10.3)	3,964 (39.8)	459 (65)	15,940 (13)	364.5 (14.6)	725.3 (41.9)	923.6 (60.4)	2,013.5 (34.9)
Provide audiometric examinations	9,613 (8.6)	3,153 (31.6)	335 (47.5)	13,100 (10.6)	292.3 (11.7)	561.9 (32.4)	620.7 (40.6)	1,474.9 (25.6)
Provide periodic pulmonary function screening	4,524 (4.0)	1,758 (17.6)	185 (26.5)	6,468 (5.3)	154.5 (6.2)	297.6 (17.2)	239.6 (15.7)	691.8 (12.0)
Provide ophthalmological examinations	11,162 (9.9)	3,293 (33.0)	371 (52.5)	14,826 (12.1)	345.8 (13.8)	596.6 (34.4)	673.6 (44)	1,616.0 (28.0)
Provide x-ray examinations	6,735 (6.0)	2,090 (21)	310 (43.9)	9,134 (7.4)	210.4 (8.4)	368.6 (21.3)	505.3 (33)	1,084.3 (18.8)
Provide periodic urine tests	4,891 (4.4)	1,291 (13)	149 (21.1)	6,331 (5.1)	160.3 (6.4)	223.9 (12.9)	301.6 (19.7)	685.8 (11.9)
Provide periodic blood tests	4,354 (3.9)	1,019 (10.2)	178 (25.2)	5,551 (4.5)	131.8 (5.3)	190 (11)	381.8 (25)	703.7 (12.2)

SOURCE: NIOSH Occupational Hazards Survey, 1977.

Table 64: Testing Regimen as Reported by Respondents in the Banking and Insurance Industries

	Percent	General Employees*	Employees in Hazardous Jobs
Testing Frequency			
Preemployment only		30%	—
Preemployment and annual		13.3	—
Annual		16.7	—
Biannual		—	—
Other (implies more often or for different groups)		30	—
Type of Tests			
Medical history	80.0		
Physical examination	66.7		
X-ray	60.0		
Pulmonary function	20.0		
Clinical laboratory	70.0		
Blood	63.3		
Urine	70.0		
Sputum	6.7		
Audiometry	20.0		
Vision tests	16.7		
EKG	46.7		
Performer of Screening			
In-house medical department	56.7		
Single outside service company	16.7		
Multiple outside providers	10.0		
All of the above	16.7		
Future Performer of Screening			
In-house resources	70.0		
Outside providers	26.7		
Special Equipment in Place			
PFT	20.0		
Audiometer	20.0		
Routine laboratory	26.7		
X-ray	30.0		
Vision	13.3		
EKG	36.7		

*In most cases only for employees older than 40 years of age.
SOURCE: F&S Survey.

Banking and Insurance. The banking and insurance industries were well represented in the F&S survey with 30 companies responding, representing more than 105,000 workers. Company size varied from 200 to 18,000 employees and there was a national representation. Physicians made up 66.7 percent of all respondents, the remainder being allied health professionals or other company personnel. Approximately 70 percent of the physicians were full-time employees and 80 percent of all companies had a full-time medical department. Only two companies did not have any screening program at all.

Screening regimens and equipment in place are shown in Table 64.

Since employees in these industries are not exposed to chemical hazards, most tests performed are those to identify early heart disease that can be easily aggravated by workplace stress. Most testing is offered to those over critical ages and it is geared to identify early signs of disease.

Estimates of the annual cost of testing per employee ranged from $25 to $200, with an average of $77.40.

The results of the F&S survey when compared with NIOSH estimates (Tables 64 and 65) show that in large plants there has been an increase in the establishment of in-house medical departments and examinations have become more extensive as they include more specialized tests. Also, a respectable number of companies responding to the F&S survey reported having a variety of medical equipment in place.

Hospital Workers. Historically, the hospital was an environment that presented certain dangers for the healthy. These dangers stemmed mainly from contagious diseases at a time when the causes of such diseases were unknown and the principles of antisepsis were still to be delineated. Even later, these principles were sometimes largely ignored. Today the dangers more often come from a kind of stress called "burn-out," or such substances as ethylene oxide used for sterilization, nitrous oxide used in anesthesia, and hexachlorophene (HCP), a widely used antibacterial agent.

The EPA has been considering banning the use of ethylene oxide in hospitals. Ethylene oxide has been found to cause sterility and chromosome damage to animals. Also suspected of causing serious health problems is HCP. The use of this substance was discontinued in hospital nurseries in 1972 when it was found to be neurotoxic to infants. Now new studies suggest that nurses exposed to this substance have greater risk of minor birth defects in their offspring. The nurses are exposed to HCP by washing their hands in detergents that contain up to 0.5% HCP.

Other potentially hazardous substances in the hospital environment are anesthetic gases that are suspected to be neurotoxic and teratogenic. Anesthetic gases escape during use in the operating rooms. The effects of anesthetic gases on hospital personnel have not been established. OSHA, however, has promulgated a new standard on nitrous oxide exposure in the hospital environment that

Table 65: Summary of Number and Percent of Plants and Employees in Plants Covered by Special Medical Services — Finance, Insurance, and Other

	Plants				Employees (thousands)			
	Small (8-99)	Medium (100-500)	Large (Over 500)	Total	Small (8-99)	Medium (100-500)	Large (Over 500)	Total
Formally established health unit	550 (1.1)	0 (0)	93 (40.4)	643 (1.2)	24 (2.2)	0 (0)	108.2 (47.8)	132.3 (6.8)
Regularly record health information about new employees	29,827 (61.3)	3,242 (89.7)	93 (40.4)	33,162 (63.2)	768.9 (70.8)	562.3 (88.7)	108.2 (47.8)	1,439.4 (74)
Require preplacement physical examinations	7,418 (15.3)	2,046 (56.6)	93 (40.4)	9,557 (18.2)	158.8 (14.6)	378.9 (59.8)	108.2 (47.8)	646 (33.2)
Provide periodic medical examinations	1,002 (2.1)	569 (15.7)	84 (36.5)	1,655 (3.2)	14.4 (1.3)	106.5 (16.8)	75.6 (33.4)	196.4 (10.1)
Provide audiometric examinations	835 (1.7)	221 (6.1)	0 (0)	1,056 (2.0)	7.5 (.7)	31.3 (4.9)	0 (0)	38.9 (2.0)
Provide periodic pulmonary function screening	0 (0)	221 (6.1)	0 (0)	221 (.4)	0 (0)	31.4 (4.9)	0 (0)	31.4 (1.6)
Provide periodic ophthalmological examinations	835 (1.7)	468 (12.9)	84 (36.5)	1,387 (2.6)	7.5 (.7)	80.8 (12.7)	75.6 (33.4)	163.9 (8.4)
Provide x-ray examinations	835 (1.7)	358 (9.9)	84 (36.5)	1,277 (2.4)	7.5 (.7)	58.8 (9.3)	75.6 (33.4)	141.9 (7.3)
Provide periodic urine tests	835 (1.7)	117 (3.2)	0 (0)	952 (1.8)	7.5 (.7)	12.9 (2.0)	0 (0)	20.4 (1.0)
Provide periodic blood tests	835 (1.7)	117 (3.2)	91 (7.3)	952 (1.8)	7.5 (.7)	12.9 (2.0)	0 (0)	20.4 (1.0)

limits the concentrations of this substance to 50 ppm. Researchers have found that in many hospitals average concentrations of this gas approach 400 ppm.

In addition to CNS effects, anesthetic gases have also been implicated in liver disease, cancer, and reproductive disorders. However, a 17-year review of deaths among anesthesiologists, carried out by the American Cancer Society, showed that anesthesiologists tend to live longer than their medical colleagues and that the causes of their deaths are similar to those of the general population. No excess of cancer deaths or deaths due to rare disorders was detected.

Approximately 23 respondents to the F&S survey were hospitals or other health facilities, with 19 being acute care hospitals. The respondents were doctors (5), registered nurses (8), and other professionals (6), responsible for overseeing 50,750 employees. As expected, 17 out of the 19 facilities had a full-time medical department with an average staff of three. Most hospitals screen their employees regularly and provide a comprehensive testing regimen, since they have the equipment and facilities in place.

Most respondents did not know the exact cost of the employee screening program. The remainder placed the costs between $15.00 and $155.00. The wide range is attributed to testing frequency per annum and the number of tests performed. Hospitals performing only one examination annually reported costs ranging between $25 and $50. Those performing biannual examinations reported annual costs nearer $155.

Special screening tests performed by the hospital not normally performed in industrial settings include: rubella titer (employees in obstetric and pediatric wards), hypertension screening, vision tests, skin, throat and nasal cultures, tuberculosis skin test (required in many states), audiometry, stool test (for food service employees), and EKG (over age 35).

The hazards encountered by hospital employees vary significantly from those in the industrial sector. Also, the problems of contracting or passing along infectious diseases is far more serious in the hospital environment than in any other workplace.

MARKET SIZE

It is extremely difficult to estimate the size of the occupational medicine market with a high degree of confidence. Although it is relatively easy to estimate the penetration of health screening with certain industries and plant sizes, it is nearly impossible to assess the impact in this field of the thousands of small plants that represent the majority of the total.

There are two separate market places within this industry; the services markets and the products markets. The former probably exhibits greater growth potential, since it offers the provider a limitless opportunity within a relatively well-defined field. The products market is highly fragmented and difficult to service.

In this section an attempt is made to estimate the services and products markets. It should be stressed that all are estimates, although based on the NIOSH and F&S surveys. Since the F&S survey provides limited information regarding current programs in plants employing fewer than 500 workers, the numbers are far more reliable for the larger plants.

Market estimates reflecting the total annual dollar value of the services performed in the industrial medicine setting are given in Table 66. Product markets are given in Table 67.

Services Markets

The services market represents a large, highly fragmented supplier group, mostly regionally oriented and serving a variety of industries and plants.

The service industry consists of the following major components:

- individual physicians (usually generalists and sometimes occupational specialists) serving industries in a highly confined regional basis.
- physician groups or hospitals serving nearby industries
- regional multisite concerns providing fixed and mobile screening services,
- national firms with extensive capabilities both in the type of medical surveillance offered and the region served, and
- highly specialized firms, such as clinical laboratories or audiometry screening specialists, which offer only selected services on a national or regional basis.

The largest group of plants (companies) is represented by those employing fewer than 100 employees. Such plants cannot afford an in-house medical department. According to the NIOSH survey, only 2.3 percent of all plants employing fewer than 100 workers had a formally established health unit and only 0.5 percent of all such plants had a physician in charge of such units. However, according to the NIOSH survey, 8.9 percent of such small plants offered periodic health examinations.

It appears that the major service provider for small plants is a physician's group, which contracts its services to neighboring industry and serves as the sole source of medical care for its employees. These services are highly regional and offer only rudiments of a comprehensive screening program. On the average, the physician spends two hours per week for each 100 workers at the plant and performs preplacement examinations in his own offices. Often he is responsible for implementing OSHA regulations and directly liable in the event of malpractice suits.

The small plant sector represents a very large and attractive market for the regional and national service provider.

The medium sized plant (100 to 500 workers) faces similar problems. Although plant size does not justify an in-house medical department, OSHA regulations regarding health screening and record keeping require that such a service be available. NIOSH estimates that in 1973 13.6 percent of all plants in this size category had a formally established health unit and 26.2 percent of such plants provided periodic health screening for their employees. The outside provider has therefore played a very important role in meeting the health-screening requirements of this plant classification.

The large sized plant (500 employees and over) is of course capable of maintaining in-house departments. Companies employing large numbers of workers with many small plants located within driving distances from each other or from a central large facility often use mobile screening units to provide on-site medical surveillance.

Mobile health screening units have a definite place in occupational medicine. They are a practical, efficient, and low cost approach to occupational screening and are currently dispatched by industry (to provide geographical coverage of several small plants) and by the service providers.

Mobile health screening vans are usually equipped to perform the following tests:

medical history (often computerized)
physical examination, such as blood pressure, temperature, neurological examination, height, weight, stethoscopic evaluation
x-ray (chest)
pulmonary function
audiometry
vision tests (tonometry, vision acuity)
EKG
sample withdrawal for blood, urine, and stool tests.

If all these examinations are performed the mobile unit can perform 15 examinations per day. If only x-rays, vision, and hearing tests are performed in addition to medical history taking and a physical examination, then the unit can perform as many as 25 tests per day.

The historic and estimated dollar value of the service component of the occupational medicine marketplace is given in Table 66. Probably 60 percent of the total sum was earned by outside consultants and most of that was paid by the small and medium sized plants. As the burden of record keeping and compliance with federal and state regulations accumulate, it is estimated that the service sector will play an increasingly important role in this market.

Table 66: Historic and Estimated Total Value of Health Screening Services in Occupational Medicine for the 1974–1989 Period ($ thousands)

Plant Size*	1974 All Industries	1974 Manufacturers	1979 All Industries	1979 Manufacturers	1984 All Industries	1984 Manufacturers	1989 All Industries	1989 Manufacturers
Small (8–99 employees)	75,048	18,008	138,540	34,302	249,381	77,958	346,356	124,731
Percent of employees screened	12.2	13	15	16.5	18	25	25	40
Medium (100–499 employees)	127,384	59,180	241,611	110,106	440,775	227,070	587,700	289,026
Percent of employees screened	29.3	32.2	37	40	45	55	60	70
Large (500 employees and over)	313,520	215,936	517,764	326,874	862,920	549,900	943,830	582,225
Percent of employees screened	64.5	75.5	72	80	80	85	85	90
Total	515,952	293,124	897,915	471,282	1,553,076	854,928	1,877,886	995,982

*Annual costs per employee are estimated as follows: $40 in 1974, $60 in 1979, $90 in 1984 and thereafter. All estimates are made in 1979 constant dollars and therefore represent real rather than inflationary growth.

SOURCE: F&S Survey.

Table 67: Historic and Estimated Dollar Markets of Medical Equipment and Devices Acquired by Industry-Based Health Departments in the 1974–1989 Period (thousands)

Plant Size*	1974 All Industries	1974 Manufacturers	1979 All Industries	1979 Manufacturers	1984 All Industries	1984 Manufacturers	1989 All Industries	1989 Manufacturers
Medium (100–499 employees)	12,000	6,000	27,232	14,504	55,964	23,460	87,092	32,416
Percent of plants	3.6	25.5	20	35	32	45	45	55
Large (500 employees and over)	3,500	500	8,696	1,352	19,040	4,640	29,384	11,228
Percent of plants	70	80.4	75	82	85	88	95	100
Total	15,500	6,500	35,928	15,856	75,004	28,100	116,476	43,644

*The value of equipment and allied products is estimated at $20,000 for medium-size plants and at $60,000 for large-size plants. Markets include both sales of new installations and replacements.

SOURCE: F&S Survey.

Products

Chapter 8 discussed in detail the kind of medical procedures and equipment commonly encountered in an occupational medicine department. Such departments can incorporate minimal equipment normally found in a generalist's office or have an exceptionally well-equipped facility with every piece of equipment imaginable from x-ray systems to computers to automated blood chemistry set-ups.

It is extremely difficult to pinpoint the type of instrumentation a facility should use based on either its size or its workplace hazards. The forecasts presented in Table 67 are based on the assumption that few if any small industries (employing fewer than 100 workers) could ever justify the purchase of specialized equipment. Also, the forecasts assume that more and more medium- and large-sized plants would establish an in-house health screening capability. The value of a set-up with minimal specialized equipment is estimated at $20,000. However, large-sized plants often incorporate equipment with a value greater than $100,000. The forecasts assume that the average large plant spends $60,000 to equip an in-house medical department.

The market figures in Table 67 also include replacements (average life-span is estimated at five years) and also equipment purchases of companies that provide contract services in this field.

MARKETING AND DISTRIBUTION STRATEGIES

Marketing in this field is complicated by the fact that the provider must approach two sources with purchasing authority; the physician and the company executive.

The company executive is the first decision maker, since he alone, perhaps out of concern for his employees or forced by OSHA regulations, makes the first step toward the implementation of a medical surveillance program. Once the company establishes such a program, the physician or other health professional heading it often has considerable decision-making power.

There are several distributors that have concentrated their efforts in this marketplace but usually sell lower cost items. Most manufacturers of equipment and devices with applications in occupational medicine have the rudiments of a specialized sales force, often consisting of a couple of salesmen based at headquarters.

Equipment is advertised in journals addressed to the occupational physician and is shown at national or regional trade shows or meetings.

Competition is intense in some markets (spirometers, audiometers) but absent in others, such as services. The best opportunities lie in this latter field.

Also, another equipment sector that appears to have an excellent long-term outlook in this market is computer systems and allied automation devices. With increasing record-keeping requirements, this industry will turn to computers to organize and maintain its data files.

Decision Makers

Occupational health screening programs vary significantly from one another, depending on the goals of the program. The primary decision maker in establishing a program is the management of each facility. The goal of the program is either to comply with federal regulations or to improve the productivity of the workers and to safeguard the health of important members of the company. Whatever the reason for the establishment of a health screening program, industry must turn to a physician for guidance in putting such a program into operation and in supervising its activities.

Once hired by a company, either on a part-time or full-time basis, the physician must decide how to implement the screening regimen required. However, does he also make the financial decisions or the purchasing decisions? The F&S survey was designed to provide an answer to this question. The results were not surprising, as can be seen in Table 68. The majority of all decisions regarding medical and scientific matters were made by physicians. However, physicians also made the majority of purchasing and financial decisions. It appears from our findings that promotion and advertising addressed to physicians is the most effective selling technique.

Several publications, such as the *Journal of Occupational Medicine, American Journal of Industrial Medicine,* and *Occupational Health & Safety*, directly address themselves to the occupational medicine specialty. However, industrial physicians also turn to a variety of medical journals to obtain up-to-date information on medical techniques covering a variety of medical conditions. For instance, a physician supervising a company medical program that leans heavily on cardiovascular screening is more likely to get his information on developments in his field from specialized journals in the cardiovascular field rather than from journals specializing in industrial medicine.

Also, since thousands of private or group practice physicians also engage in occupational medicine through their office practice but do not consider themselves occupational specialists, it is essential that product and service providers use a more diverse forum to display their capabilities. For instance, it would be helpful if a display of a new EKG presented at an exhibit that is a part of a cardiologists' convention included special information and data on the product's application possibilities in occupational medicine.

Table 68: Decision Makers in the Operation of a Company Screening Program

Decision Makers	Purchasing	Medical	Scientific	Financial
Physician	43.6	67.7	53.9	41.9
Nurse	19.7	14.8	7.2	7.4
Purchasing Department	4.5	0.4	4.1	4.1
Administration	11.1	1.4	3.0	9.4
Company management	8.6	3.9	13.3	22.6
Safety director	4.1	2.0	3.9	4.1
Other	8.4	9.8	14.6	10.5

SOURCE: F&S Survey.

10
Suppliers of Products and Services

The list of the major suppliers of specialized equipment and services in the occupational medicine field represent those that have directly advertised in journals addressed to the occupational physician or have displayed their products in occupational medicine exhibits.

Nearly every maker of medical products might sell products that have an application in occupational medicine. However, there are many suppliers that have concentrated some effort in marketing specifically in this field and these stand to capture the bulk of the business.

Unlike product makers, service providers are few and have highly targeted marketing programs. Most of the ones listed are national in scope and have a multisite capability using both fixed and mobile units. There are numerous regional providers also (see Appendix C) but these do not compete on a large scale. Finally, many hospitals are also entering this market. The ones with an excellent outlook are those that belong to national chains that can offer the service at multiple locations on a national basis.

Table 69: Product Manufacturers

Company	Product
Air Shields, Inc. 330 Jacksonville Rd. Halboro, PA 19040 Tel: (215) 675-5200	Vitalor Pulmonary Function Testing System
American Cystoscope Makers, Inc. 300 Stillwater Ave. Stamford, CT 06902 Tel: (203) 357-8300	Flexible Fiberoptic Endoscopes
American Monitor Corporation Box 68505 Indianapolis, IN 46268 Tel: (317) 297-4100	Clinical Laboratory Analyzers
American Optical Medical Division Crosby Drive Bedford, MA 01730 Tel: (617) 275-0500	Vision Testing Equipment
Applied Medical Research 5041 West Cypress Str. Tampa, FL 33607 Tel: (813) 870-0003	Autoscreen Blood Pressure Screening Automatic Pressure & Heart Rate
Argosy Manufacturing Co. 60 Vista Rd. Versailles, OH 45380 Tel: (513) 526-3131	Mobil Audiometer Test Center
Audiometer Corporation of America Phoenix, AZ 85021 Tel: (602) 995-1441	The Besserman "Automated Manual" Audiometer & Data Management System
AVIV Associates 810 Towbin Ave. Lakewood, NJ 08701 Tel: (201) 367-1663	Hematofluorometer
Bausch & Lomb One Lincoln First Square Rochester, NY 14601 Tel: (716) 338-6000	Vision Testing Systems

Table 69: continued

Company	Product
Beltone Electronics Corp. Hearing Test Instrument Division 4201 W. Victoria Chicago, IL 60646 Tel: (312) 583-3600	Audiometer Model 109 Sound Booths
Breon Laboratories Instrument & Life Support Div. 90 Park Ave. New York, NY 10016 Tel: (212) 972-4141	Model 2400 Spirometer
Buchler Instruments, Inc. 1327 Sixteenth Str. Fort Lee, NJ 07024 Tel: (201) 224-3333	Portable Fluorometer to Measure ZPP
The Burdick Corporation 15 Plumb Str. Milton, WI 53563 Tel: (800) 356-0701	EKG
Cambridge Instruments Co. 73 Spring Str. Ossining, NY 10562 Tel: (914) 941-8100	EKG Stress Test System
Cardio-Pulmonary Instruments, Inc. 6400 Westpark Street Houston, TX 77036 Tel: (713) 783-7520	Spirometers, Gas Analyzers
Cavitron Cardiopulmonary Sales 270 E. Palais Rd. Anaheim, CA 92805 Tel: (714) 776-1811/(800) 854-3894	SC-20 Spirometric Computer Donti Pulmonary Performance Analyzer
CDx, Inc. 10691 E. Bethany Drive Aurora, CO 80014 Tel: (800) 525-3515	CDx Pulmonary Analyzer

(Table 69: continued overleaf)

Table 69: continued

Company	Product
Warren E. Collins, Inc. 220 Wood Rd. Braintree, MA 02184 Tel: (617) 383-0028	Spirometry Microprocessor, Spirometer (FVC, FEV_T, FEV_T/FVC%, $FeF_{25-75\%}$, IVC & MVV)
Digilab, Inc. 237 Putnam Ave. Cambridge, MA 02139 Tel: (617) 868-4330	Intraocular Pressure & Pulse Measuring Instrument
Dyna Med 6200 Yarrow Dr. Carlsbad, CA 92008 Tel: (714) 438-2511	Hare-Elder Demand Valve/ Rescuscitator
Eckel Industries Eckoustic Div. 155 Fawcett Str. Cambridge, MA 02138 Tel: (617) 491-3221	Audiometric Examination Booths, Rooms & Suites
Environmental Technology Corp. 30405 Solon Rd. Cleveland, OH 44139 Tel: (216) 248-2250	Microprocessor/Spirometer with Optional RS-232 Computer Interface (FVC, FEV, percent of normal FVC & FEV & FEV_1/FVC)
ESA Environmental Sciences Assoc., Inc. 45 Wiggins Ave. Bedford, MA 01730 Tel: (617) 275-0100	Model 4000 Hematofluorometer for zinc protoporphyrin & Blood Lead Measurements, Model 3010A Trace Metals Analyzer (direct blood lead measurements)
Genie Audio, Inc. 9679 Peloquin Montreal, Canada H2C 2J4 Tel: (514) 388-9212	Automatic Hearing Loss Audiometer
George Koch Sons, Inc. Thermal Acoustics Div. 2112 Pennsylvania Ave. Evansville, IN 47744 Tel: (812) 426-9759	Audiometric Booths

Table 69: continued

Company	Product
Grayson Stadler, Inc. 537 Great Rd. Littleton, MA 01460 Tel: (617) 486-3514	Automatic Recording

Gulf & Western Applied Sciences Labs
Gulf & Western Research &
  Development Group
335 Bear Hill Rd.
Waltham, MA 02154
Tel: (617) 890-5100
	Real Time Pulse & ECG Rate
	  Measurement Instrument
	  (Battery Operated)

Industrial Acoustics Co. 1160 Commerce Ave. Bronx, NY 10462 Tel: (212) 931-8000	Audiometric Test Rooms
IPCO Medical Instrument Div. 1025 Westchester Ave. White Plains, NY 10604 Tel: (914) 682-4570	Portable Defibrillator
Jobst Institute, Inc. Box 653 Toledo, OH 43694 Tel: (419) 698-1611	Anti/Shock Air Pants
Jones Medical Instrument Co. 200 Windsor Drive Oak Brook, IL 60521 Tel: (312) 654-1980	Pulmonor II Spirometer
Keystone View Division of Mast Development Co. 2212 E. 12th Str. Davenport, IA 52803 Tel: (319) 326-0141	Vision Screening System

(Table 69: continued overleaf)

Table 69: continued

Company	Product
LSE Corporation 6 Gill Street Woburn, MA 01801 Tel: (617) 935-4954	Portable, Fully Preprogrammed Vanguard Computerized Spirometer (PEF, FVC, FEV_1, $FEV_{1\%}$, MVV TV measured, and FVC, FEV_1, $FEV_{1\%}$, FEF_{25-75} MVV Predicted)
Maico Hearing Instruments, Inc. 7375 Bush Lake Rd. Minneapolis, MN 55435 Tel: (612) 835-4400	Computer Audiometer with Automatic Printout
Marion Health & Safety, Inc. Dept. OHS-979 9233 Ward Parkway Kansas City, MO 64114 Tel: (800) 821-5502/(816) 361-0048	Uni-Flex Institutional Pak (medicine, first aid, dermatological emergency products)
National Draeger, Inc. 401 Parkway View Drive Pittsburgh, PA 15205 Tel: (412) 787-1131	Alcohol Testing Kit Co Breath Kit
Ohio Medical Products, Division of Airco 3030 Airco Dr. P.O. Box 1319 Madison, WI 53707 Tel: (608) 221-1551	Ohio 822 Spirometer
Park Surgical Co., Inc. 5001 New Utrecht Ave. Brooklyn, NY 11219 Tel: (212) 436-9200	Goodlite Vision Acuity Testing
Physio-Control 11811 Willows Rd. Redmond, WA 98052 Tel: (206) 883-1181	Portable Defibrillators
Picker Corporation 595 Miner Rd. Highland Heights, OH 44143 Tel: (216) 449-3000	Clinex-C, Low Cost Chest X-ray Systems

Table 69: continued

Company	Product
Reedco, Inc. P.O. Box 345, 54 E. Genesee Str. Auburn, NY 13021 Tel: (315) 252-0020	Arthroidial Protractor for Measurement of Body Joint Motion
Smith Kline Diagnostics P.O. Box 1947 Sunnyvale, CA 94086 Tel: (408) 732-6000	Homoccult Booth for test of fecal occult blood
Smith & Wesson 2100 Roosevelt Ave. Springfield, MA 01101 Tel: (413) 781-8300	Breathalyzer Model 1000 for alcohol detection
SRL Medical 2676 Indian Riffle Road Dayton, OH 45440 Tel: (513) 426-0033	Automated Pulmonary Function Lab Model 220 Dry Rolling Seal Spirometer
Titmus Optical, Inc. Protective Products Div. P.O. Box 191 Petersburg, VA 23803 Tel: (800) 446-1802	Vision Testing Equipment to Measure Visual Skills
Tracor, Inc. Medical Instrument Div. 6500 Tracor Lane Austin, TX 78721 Tel: (800) 423-2355/ (512) 926-2800	Hearing Conservation Programs, Audiometric Booths, Microprocessor Audiometer with Permanent Record
Vital Assists, Inc. 4100 E. Dry Creek Rd. Littleton, CO 80122 Tel: (303) 770-2700	Pulmonary Function Analyzer
Vitalograph Medical Instrumentation 8347 Quivira Rd. Lenexa, KS 66215 Tel: (913) 888-4221/ (800) 255-6626	Spirometers

Table 70: Service Providers

Company	Services
American Biomedical Corporation 1525 Viceroy, Suite 300 Dallas, TX 75235	Medical Surveillance Program
Bio-Science Laboratories Van Nuys, CA 91409 Tel: (213) 989-2520	Clinical Laboratory
Cameron Medical Corporation 2716 E. Florence Ave. Huntington Park, CA 90255 Tel: (213) 588-1201	Medical Supplier
Cyber Diagnostics, Inc. 3600 S. Yosemite, Suite 530 Denver, CO 80237 Tel: (303) 779-3690	Pulmonary Function Testing Using Portable Acquisition Systems
Damon Medical Laboratories 115 Fourth Ave. Needham Heights, MA 02194 Tel: (617) 449-3120	Clinical Laboratory
Diamond Shamrock Health Systems 111 Superior Ave. Cleveland, OH 44114 Tel: (216) 694-6242	Mobile & Fixed Site, Health Date Collection (COHESS-Computerized Occupational Health Environmental Surveillance System)
Enbionics (A Metpath Co.) 1469 South Holly Str. Denver, Co. 80222 Tel: (303) 758-0430	Health/Environmental/Toxicology Consulting & Testing Services
Environmental Sciences Associates, Inc. 45 Wiggins Ave. Bedford, MA 01746 Tel: (617) 275-0100	Lead and Other Metal Exposure Monitoring
Health Evaluation Programs, Inc. 808 Busse Highway Park Ridge, IL 60068 Tel: (312) 696-1824	Mobil Health Screening Service

Table 70: continued

Company	Services
Hearex Occupational Health Services A Subsidiary of Kemper Corp. P.O. Box 18425 Tampa, FL 33679 Tel: (813) 251-8491	Health Screening & Data Collection
HSC Services, Inc. 1660 S. Albion St. Suite 619 Denver, CO 80222 Tel: (303) 757-7409	Injury/Illness Trend Reporting
ICN Medical Laboratories, Inc. 6060 N.E. 112th Ave. Portland, OR 97208 Tel: (503) 255-1220	Pre-employment Screens
Keltron Corporation 225 Crescent Str. Waltham, MA 02154 Tel: (617) 894-8700	Automated Interview/Medical History
Laboratory Services 150 S. Autumn Str. San Jose, CA 95110 Tel: (408) 288-9850	Clinical Laboratory
Mediscan 172 N. Tustin Orange, CA 92667 Tel: (714) 997-3060	On-site Multiphasic Health Tests
Metpath 60 Commerce Way Hackensack, NJ 07606 Tel: (201) 288-0900	Epidemiological Surveillance and Clinical Laboratory
Micronetic Laboratories 1688 Willow St. San Jose, CA 95125 Tel: (408) 265-3500	Sputum Cytology

(Table 70: continued overleaf)

Table 70: continued

Company	Services
Mobilhealth Detection Office, Inc. 8B 20 South Str. Morristown, NJ 07960 Tel: (201) 267-5938	Mobile Health Testing
Pacific Southwest Medical Group Urvine, CA Tel: (714) 557-8820	Medical & Hygiene Services
Parasitology Laboratory of Washington 2141 K. Street, N.W., Suite 500 Washington, DC 20037 Tel: (202) 331-0287	Diagnostic Parasitology Lab
Phone-A-Gram System, Inc. One S. Park San Francisco, CA 94107 Tel: (415) 433-4170	Computerized Electrocardiogram
Physical Measurements, Inc. P.O. Box 4081 Atlanta, GA 30302 Tel: (404) 952-9997	Mobile Health Testing (blood pressure, tonometry, x-ray, EKG, PFT, blood & urine)
Professional Health Services, Inc. 83. S. Eagle Rd. Havertown, PA 19083 Tel: (215) 853-1330	Mobile Multi-phasic Industrial Health Testing
ToxiGenics, Inc. 1800 E. Pershing Rd. Decatur, IL 62526 Tel: (217) 875-3930	Toxicological Analysis of Biological Samples
TRC, The Research Group Corp. of New England 125 Silas Deane Highway Wethersfield, CT 06109 Tel: (203) 563-1431	Toxic Exposure Data Program
UBTL Division University of Utah Research Institute 520 Wahara Way Salt Lake City, UT 84108 Tel: (801) 581-8183	Toxicological Analysis of Biological Samples

Appendixes

Appendix A
Regional Offices of OSHA

REGION I (CT, MA, ME, NH, RI, VT)
16 North Street
Boston, MA 02109
Telephone: (617) 223-6710

REGION II (NJ, NY, PR, VI, CZ)
Room 3445, 1 Astor Plaza
1515 Broadway
New York, NY 10036
Telephone: (212) 944-3426

REGION III (DC, DE, MD, PA, VA, WV)
Gateway Building, Suite 2100
3535 Market Street
Philadelphia, PA 19104
Telephone: (215) 596-1201

REGION IV (AL, FL, GA, KY, MS, NC, SC, TN)
1375 Peachtree Street, N.E.
Suite 587
Atlanta, GA 30367
Telephone: (404) 881-3573

REGION V (IL, IN, MI, MN, OH, WI)
230 South Dearborn Street
32nd Floor, Room 3230
Chicago, IL 60604
Telephone: (312) 353-2220

REGION VI (AR, LA, NM, OK, TX)
555 Griffin Square Bldg., Room 602
Dallas, TX 75202
Telephone: (214) 767-4731

REGION VII (IA, KS, MO, NE)
911 Walnut Street, Room 3000
Kansas City, MO 64106
Telephone: (816) 374-5861

REGION VIII (CO, MT, ND, SD, UT, WY)
Federal Bldg., Room 1554
1961 Stout Street
Denver, CO 80294
Telephone: (303) 837-5285

REGION IX (AZ, CA, HI, NV)
Box 36017
450 Golden Gate Ave.
San Francisco, CA 94102
Telephone: (415) 556-0584

REGION X (AK, ID, OR, WA)
Federal Office Bldg., Room 6003
909 First Avenue
Seattle, WA 98174
Telephone: (206) 442-5930

Appendix B
Frost & Sullivan Occupational Medicine Questionnaire

1. What is the chief product manufactured by your Company (plant)?
   Product _____
   # of employees involved _____
2. Please describe your job capacity
   Industrial Physician _____ Industrial Hygienist _____ R.N. _____
   Part time _____
   Full time _____
3. Does your Company, plant or division have a full time medical department?
   Yes _____ No _____
   If yes, how many workers are supervised? _____
       how many professionals are employed? _____
   If no, who is responsible for implementing the medical aspects PL 91-596? _____
4. How often do you screen:
   general employees?
       pre-employment only _____
       annually _____
       biannually _____
       other _____
   employees in hazardous jobs?
       pre-employment only _____
       annually _____
       biannually _____
       other _____

5. What tests are performed in a standard (non complaint-related) screening procedure?

    ____ medical history   ____ clinical laboratory
    ____ physical examination   ____ urine
    ____ X-ray   ____ blood
    ____ other (please list)   ____ sputum
                                          ____ other (please list)

6. Who performs the medical screening in your facility?

    Company medical department _____
    Single outside service company _____
    Multiple outside providers _____
    All of the above _____ (in this case please rank 1, 2, 3)

7. In the future do you expect to do most of the screening using

    in-house resources _____
    outside providers _____

8. What medical equipment is currently available to perform in-house tests? (Please list)

    _____
    _____

9. What is the average annual cost of the medical screening program per employee? _____

10. Do you expect the average cost to rise in the future?

Year	Cost ($)
1980	_____
1985	_____

11. What developments in the medical equipment, supplies and services areas would you encourage to aid you in your practice?

    _____
    _____

12. In your department who makes

    the purchasing decisions   _____
    the medical decisions   _____
    the financial decisions   _____
    the scientific decisions   _____

13. Do you believe that a regular medical screening regimen is necessary to protect the health of the industrial worker?

    _____
    _____

Appendix B   219

14. Do you foresee that such a regimen would be required by law? _____
    _____

15. What type of screening would you recommend in the area you specifically supervise and/or perform research in?
    area of expertise _____

Test	Frequency
_____	_____
_____	_____
_____	_____
_____	_____
_____	_____
_____	_____

16. Is preventive medicine a workable concept in your area?
    Yes _____   No _____
    Please, comment _____

17. Would an on-site multiphasic screening installation benefit your program and be cost effective?
    Yes _____   No _____
    Please, comment _____
    _____

18. Are you satisfied with the current federal regulations in this field?
    Yes _____   No _____
    Please, comment _____
    _____

19. Do you think that a mandatory, periodic, medical mass screening program of industrial workers would:

	Yes	No
prevent occupationally induced diseases	_____	_____
improve the health outlook of the workers	_____	_____
be cost effective	_____	_____
jeopardize the privacy of workers	_____	_____
increase the cost of medical care without providing any real benefits	_____	_____

    Other (please explain) _____
    _____

20. Thank you very much for your help. Would you be available for a personal _____ or telephone _____ interview?

Appendix C
List of Companies and Institutions that Have Contributed to the Survey

Users

Abbott Laboratories
Abex Corporation (2 facilities)
Abu-Garcia, Inc.
Airsearch Manufacturing Corp.
 of Arizona
Alcoa (4 facilities)
Alliance of America Insurers
Allied Chemical (2 facilities)
American Can Corporation
American Cyanamid Company
 (4 facilities)
American International Group
 (2 facilities)
American Mutual Insurance Company
American Tobacco Company
Amerock Corporation
A. O. Smith Corporation
Armco, Inc. (2 facilities)
Arthur D. Little, Inc.
Asarco
Atlantic Research Corporation
AT & T (3 facilities)
Aztec
Babcock & Wilcox
Baltimore City Hospital

Baltimore Gas & Electric
Basic, Inc.
Battelle Memorial Institute
Bell Telephone Labs.
Bethlehem Steel
Bituminous Insurance Companies
Boise Cascade Corporation
Borden Thermoplastics
Boston Edison Company
Brookline, Town of
Brush Wellman, Inc.
Bucyrus Erie
Buick Motor Division
Bureau of National Affairs, Inc.
Burlington Industries (2 locations)
Burroughs Corporation (2 locations)
California Institute of Technology
 Caltech
California State Compensation Insurance
 Fund
Campbell Soup Company
Cannon Mills Company
Carborundum Company
Caterpillar Tractor Co. (3 locations)
C-E Air Preheater Company

Center for Toxicology Man & Environment, Inc.
Century Brass Products, Inc.
C & H Sugar Company
Champlin Petroleum
Chesebrough-Ponds, Inc.
Chrysler Corporation
Ciba Geigy Pharmaceuticals
CIT Financial Corporation
Citibank
Clark Equipment Company
Clark Grane Vault Company
Clay Equipment Corporation
Colt Industries (2 facilities)
Columbus & Southern Ohio Electric Co.
Commonwealth Edison Corporation
Communications Satellite Corporation
Community Hospital at the Monterey Pen.
Connecticut Gas Supply Corporation
Connecticut General Life Insurance Co.
Connecticut Mutual Life Insurance Co.
Conoco
Consolidated Bio Medical Labs., Inc.
Continental Bank
Continental Can Company
Contra Cost County Health Department
Cook County Hospital
Coors Industries, Inc.
Copland Corporation
Cornell University Medical College
Corpus Christi, City of
Courtaulds North America, Inc.
C+P Telephone Company
Crown Central Petroleum Company
Cuna Mutual Insurance Group
Dan River Inc.
Dariron Co., Inc.
Dravo Corporation (2 facilities)
Department of the Army
Denver, City & County of
Diamond Shamrock Corporation
Dillingham Maritime Pacific Div.
Dillingham Ship Repair

Documation
Dow Corning Corporation
Dow Chemical Co. (6 facilities)
DWP R.R.
Eastman Kodak Co. (2 facilities)
Eastern Virginia Medical School
Eaton Corp., Euclid Clinic Foundation
EG&G
E. I. Dupont (7 facilities)
Eli Lilly & Company
Emerson Hospital
Employees Insurance of Wausau (2 locations)
EPA (2 facilities)
E. R. Squibb & Sons, Inc.
ESB Ray-O-Vac
East Side Occupational Health Center
European Motors, Inc.
Exxon Company (2 facilities)
FAA (2 facilities)
Fairfield Mfg. Co., Inc.
Fairfax County Health Department
Federal Cartridge Corporation
Fermilab
Firestone Tire & Rubber Co.
First Wisc. National Bank
Fisherbody Division G.M.C. (4 locations)
Ford Aerospace & Comm. Corp.
Ford Motor Co. (3 facilities)
Fruehauf Corporation
General Electric (8 facilities)
General Foods
General Motors Corp. (4 locations)
General Telephone Co. of Indiana
Gillette Company
Goodwill Industries, Inc.
Gould, Inc.
Gray Tool Company
Great Lakes Steel
Great Northern Paper Company
Grumman Aerospace (2 facilities)
GTE Sylvania

Appendix C

Gulf & Western
Gulf Oil Corporation
Hartford Insurance Group
Harvard University
Harvey's Wagon Wheel, Inc.
Hawaiian Telephone Co.
Hesston, Inc.
Hoffmann-La Roche, Inc.
Homestake Mining Co.
Honeywell, Inc. (2 facilities)
Hooker Chemical Co. (2 facilities)
Hughes Aircraft Co.
Hughes Air West
Huntington Memorial Hospital
IBM Corporation
ICI Americas, Inc.
Indiana Bell Telephone Co., Inc.
Ingersoll-Rand Co. (2 facilities)
Instrumentation Lab., Inc.
Insurance Company of North America
International Harvester (2 facilities)
International Paper Co.
ITT Nesbitt
James River Graphics, Inc.
John Deere Company
John Hancock Mutual Life Ins. Co.
Johnson Controls, Inc.
J. R. Simplot Company
J. T. Baker Chemical Company
Kaiser Aluminum Corporation
Kay Fries, Inc.
Kelly-Springfield Tire Company
Kimberly Clark (2 facilities)
Knott's Berry Farm
Kollsman Instrument Company
Lamson Division
Lawyers Cooperative
Liberty Mutual Insurance Co.
Litton Industries
Lord Corporation
Los Angeles, City of
Los Angeles, County of (2 facilities)
Maricopa County General Hospital

Marsh Instrument Company
Maryland Casualty Company
Martin Marietta
McCord Corporation
McNeil Labs
Metalbestos Systems
Miners Rocks Ind. Enterprises
Mountain Bell (2 locations)
Mount Sinai Medical Center
National Health Watch, Inc.
Nationwide Insurance Company
Naval Hospital
Naval Medical Research Institute
Naval Regional Medical Center
 (3 facilities)
Naval Undersea Medical Institute
Navy Environmental Health Center
New York Hospital-Cornell Med. Center
New York Life Insurance Company
New York Telephone Co. (2 facilities)
NIOSH (3 facilities)
Norfolk Shipbuilding & Dry Dock Co.
Northeastern Electric System
Northern State Power Company
Northwestern Bell Telephone Co.
Olin Corporation (2 locations)
OSHA (3 facilities)
Otis Engineering Corporation
Pacific Mutual Life Insurance Co.
Pacific Telephone Co. (3 facilities)
Pan American World Airways
Park Enterprises
Penna Mfg. Assoc. Insurance Co.
P & G
Potlatch Company
Pratt & Lamburg, Inc.
Pratt & Whitney
Presbyterian Hospital
PRI
Princeton University
Proctor & Gamble Company
Providence Medical Center
P. R. Mallory Company, Inc.

Prudential Company of America
Prupac
Puget Sound Naval Shipyard
Public Health Service
Radian Corporation
Raybestos Friction Materials
RCA
Remington Arms Company, Inc.
Republic Steel (3 locations)
Reynolds Electric & Engineering Co.
Reynolds Metal Co. (2 facilities)
Rhinelander Paper Company
Rhode Island Dept. of Health
Riverview Hospital
Rockwell International (2 facilities)
R. R. Donneley & Sons Company
Russell Stover
Safeway Stores, Inc.
Saginaw Steering Gears
Salt River Project
San Bernardino County
San Diego, City of
Santa Ana Tustin Community Hospital
Scott Paper Company
Sears Roebuck & Co. (2 facilities)
Shell Development Corporation
Shell Oil
Singer Company
South Carolina Dept. of Health
South Central Bell
Southeastern Program Center Service
Southern Pacific Transportation Co.
Southern Railway Company
Southland Corporation
Southwestern Bell Telephone Co.
Southwire Company
Sperry Rand Company
Sperry Univac
Spring Mills, Inc.
St. Agnes Health Appraisal
Standard Oil Company (Ohio)
St. Anthony Hospital
Standard Oil Industries

St. Elizabeth Hospital
Stewart Warner
St. Joseph Hospital, Omaha, Neb.
St. Joseph Hospital, Fort Wayne, Ind.
St. Joseph Medical Association
St. Vincent Hospital
Suffolk County Government
Sun Ship Building & Dry Dock Co.
Sun Petroleum Products Company
Syntex
Technicon Instruments Corporation
Teledyne Wah Chang Albany
Tenneco Chemicals, Inc.
Texaco, Inc.
Textron, Inc. (2 facilities)
TRW-Geometer Tool
Twin Cities Army Ammunition Plant
Uniformed Services Univ. (2 facilities)
Union Carbide Corporation (3 locations)
University of Chicago Hospital
University of Florida
University of Hawaii
University of Rochester
University of South Florida
University of Southern California
Univ. of Tennessee-College of Pharmacy
University of Texas
University of Vermont
U.S.A. Meddac
U.S. Air Force
U.S. Assay Office
U.S. Coast Guard
U.S. Department of Commerce-NBS
U.S. Navy Environmental & Preventive Med.
U.S. Navy Pacific Missile Test Center
U.S. Navy Portsmouth Naval Shipyard (N.H.)
U.S. Navy Shipyard-Norfolk
U.S. Post Office
U.S.S. Nimitz
U.S. Steel (5 facilities)
Virginia Chemicals, Inc.

VVP
Western Electric (6 facilities)
Western Union
Westinghouse (3 facilities)
Westvaco Corp.-Kraft Division
Weyerhouser Company
Whirlpool Corporation

The Williams Company
Wilmington Medical Center
Wisconsin Steel
West Virginia University Med. Center
Zenith (2 facilities)
Zidell Exp

Service Providers
Burbank Medical Clinic
City Public Service
East Range Clinics, Ltd.
Environ Health Associates
Equitable Environmental Health, Inc.
Executive Health Examiners Group
Grand Rapids Occupational Medicine
Grants Clinic
Harcout Clume, Inc.
Houstonian Preventive Medicine Center
Industrial Health Services
Institute of Preventive Medicine
Jackson Clinic
JRB Associates, Inc.
Kimbro Clinic Associates

Life Extension Institute
Medical Screening Clinic
Medical & Surgical Clinic S.C.
Multi-Phasic Health Systems, Inc.
Neilson Associates
Paternostro-Boyd Clinic
Peterson Associates
Physicians Associates, Chartered
Pittsburgh Diagnostic Clinic
Preventive Med. Institute/Strang Clinic
Raymond A. Yerg & Associates
R. I. Group Health Associates
Valley Primary Health Care & Preventive
 Medicine

Bibliography

1. Abrams, Herbert L., *The Overutilization of X-rays*, New England Journal of Medicine, Vol. 300, #21, May 24, 1979.
2. Alexander, Tom, *OSHA's Ill-Conceived Crusade Against Cancer*, Fortune, July 3, 1978.
3. Blair, Aaron & Fraumeni, Joseph F., *Geographic Patterns of Bladder Cancer in the United States*, J. Natl. Cancer Inst., Vol. 61, #6, December 1978.
4. Blot, William J. & Fraumeni, Joseph F., *Geographic Patterns of Bladder Cancer in the U.S.*, J. Natl. Cancer Inst., Vol. 61, #4, October 1978.
5. Blot, William J. & Fraumeni, Joseph F., *Geographic Patterns of Oral Cancer in the United States: Etiologic Implications*, Journal of Chronic Diseases, Vol. 30, 1977.
6. Blot, William J., et al., *Cancer Mortality in U.S. Counties with Petroleum Industries*, Science, Vol. 198, October 7, 1977.
7. Blot, William J., et al. *Geographic Correlates of Pancreas Cancer in the United States*, Cancer #1, Vol. 42, July 1978.
8. Breslow, Lester & Somers, Annie R., *The Lifetime Health-Monitoring Program*, The New England Journal of Medicine, Vol. 296, #11, March 17, 1977.
9. Brinton, Louise A., et al., *A Death Certificate Analysis of Nasal Cancer Among Furniture Workers in North Carolina*, Cancer Research, Vol. 37, October 1977.
10. Bronson, Gail, *Cancer Cases Spark Concern About Radiation; Scientists Debate 'Safe' Limit for U.S. Workers*, Wall Street Journal, Nov. 7, 1978.
11. Brownson, P.J. & Olson, R.J., *Using Computers to Promote Health & Safety*, Occupational Health & Safety, 48:13C May/June 1979.
12. Buchan, R.M. & Majestic, J.R., *Delivering Health Services to Small Industry in Colorado*, Occupational Health & Safety 48:42 September 1979.

13. Bylinsky, Gene, *A New Power To Predict-And Prevent Disease*, Fortune, September 25, 1978.
14. *Carcinogens*, Department of Labor, OSHA The Federal Register, Vol. 39, #20, Part III, January 29, 1974.
15. Carlson, Watter, S., et al., *Instrumentation For Measurement of Sensory Loss In The Fingertips*, Journal of Occupational Medicine, Vol. 21, #4, April 1979.
16. Claiborne, Robert, *A Penny of Prevention: The Cure For America's Health Care System*, Saturday Review, January 6, 1979.
17. *The Controversy Over the Health Effects of Radiation*, Najarian, Thomas, Technology Review, November 1978.
18. *A Cross-Sectional Epidemiologic Survey of Vinyl Chloride Workers*, NIOSH, June 1977.
19. Deletes, Roger, *The Need for Epidemiologists*, JAMA, Vol. 242, #15, October 12, 1979.
20. Elliott, John, *Escaping Anesthetic Gases May Affect Neurophysiological Functions*, JAMA, Vol. 240, #18, October 27, 1978.
21. *Etiology Vague? Probe The Work History*, Patient Care, February 28, 1979.
22. Feldman, Robert G., *Urban Lead Mining: Lead Intoxication Among Deleaders*, New England Journal of Medicine, Vol. 298, #20, May 18, 1978.
23. Fielding, Jonathan E., *Preventive Medicine & the Bottom Line*, Journal of Occupational Medicine, Vol. 21, #2, February 1979.
24. *Fitting The Workplace Into The Workup*, Patient Care, October 15, 1978.
25. Fraumeni, Joseph F., & Blot William J., *Geographic Variation In Esophageal Cancer Mortality In The United States*, Journal of Chronic Diseases, Vol. 30, 1977.
26. Gallagher, Michael, *Innovative Services Save Industrial Time Loss*, Occupational Health & Safety, 48:46, Sept. 1979.
27. *A Guide to Procedures of the Occupational Safety & Health Review Commission*; OSHA, Revised 1978.
28. *Guide to Small Plant Occupational Health Programs*, American Medical Association, 1973.
29. *Guide Lines for use of Routine X-Ray Examinations in Occupational Medicine*, Journal of Occupational Medicine, Vol. 21, #7, July 1979.
30. Haas, Joanna F. & Schotienfeld, David, *Risks of the Offspring from Parental Exposures*, Journal of Occupational Medicine, Vol. 21, #9, Sept. 1979.
31. Hanis, Nancy M., et al., *Cancer Mortality in Oil Refinery Workers*, Journal of Occupational Medicine, Vol. 21, #3, March 1979.
32. Hetu, Raymond, *Critical Analysis of the Effectiveness Of Secondary Prevention Of Occupational Hearing Loss*, Journal of Occupational Medicine, Vol. 21, #4, April 1979.
33. Hogstedt, Christer, et al., *Leukemia in Workers Exposed to Ethylene Oxide*, JAMA, Vol. 241, #11, March 16, 1979.
34. Hudson, Richard L., *Hazardous Duty: Lack of Medical Staff Heightens Health Peril in Some Small Plants*. Wall Street Journal, April 20, 1979.
35. *Is Spirometry Practical in Your Office?* Patient Care, October 15, 1978.

36. Lebowitz, Michael D., et al., *Pulmonary Function in Smelter Workers*, Journal of Occupational Medicine, Vol. 21, # 4, April 1979.
37. Lyon, Joseph L., et al., *Childhood Leukemia Associated with Fallout from Nuclear Testing*, New England Journal of Medicine, Vol. 300, # 8, February 22, 1978.
38. Meyer, C. R. & Sutherland, H. C., Jr., *A Technique for Totally Automated Audiometry*, IEEE Transactions on Biomedical Engineering, March 1976.
39. Milham, Samuel, Jr., *Mortality in Aluminum Reduction Plant Workers*, Journal of Occupational Medicine, Vol. 21, # 7, July 1979.
40. Murray, Thomas, *The Heyday of the Testing Labs*, Dun's Review, August, 1978.
41. Najarian, Thomas, *The Controversy Over the Health Effects of Radiation*, Technology Review, November 1978.
42. *National Occupational Hazards Survey*, Vol. III, NIOSH, HEW, 1977.
43. *A National Survey of the Occupational Safety & Health Work Force*, NIOSH, DHEW, July 1978.
44. *OSHA Handbook For Small Businesses*, U.S. Department of Labor, OSHA, Revised 1977.
45. Pearson, John R., *Devising Your Own Surveillance Program*, Occupational Health & Safety, May/June 1979.
46. *Physicians' Guide to the Occupational Safety & Health Act Of 1970*, Council on Occupational Health, JAMA, Vol. 219, February 14, 1972.
47. *Pointers For Detecting Hearing Loss*, Patient Care, August 15, 1977.
48. *Public Law 91–596*, 91st Congress, S. 2193, December 29, 1970.
49. Reddig, William, *Industry's Pre-Emptive Strike Against Cancer*, Fortune, Feb. 13, 1978.
50. *A Retrospective Survey of Cancer in Relation to Occupation*; U.S. DHEW, Public Health Service, Center for Disease Control, NIOSH, 1977.
51. Rom, William N., *Medicine Re-Enters the Workplace*; The New England Journal of Medicine, Vol. 300, # 12, March 22, 1979.
52. Ryan, Eugene J., *Implementing Health Services for Small Businesses*, Occupational Health & Safety, 48:16, July/August 1979.
53. Sheps, Samuel B., et al., *Utilization of the Pre-Employment Health Examination in a University Staff Health Service*, Journal of Occupational Medicine, Vol. 21, # 7, July 1979.
54. *A Shift to Common Sense Priorities*, OSHA 1977.
55. Strasser, Alexander L., *Dermatitis: An Occupational Physician's Dilemma*, Occupational Health & Safety, 48:14, May/June 1979.
56. Strasser, Alexander L., *Pre-Placement Screening: An Exercise In Preventive Medicine*, Occupational Health & Safety, 48:23, July/August 1979.
57. *Summary of NIOSH Recommendations for Occupational Health Standards*, DHEW, PHS, CDC, NIOSH, October 1978.
58. Tsai, M. J., et al., *Automatic Classification of Spirometric Data*, IEEE Transactions on Biomedical Engineering, Vol. BME-26, # 5, May 1979.
59. Wasserman, D., et al., *A Very Versatile Simultaneous Multifinger Photocell Plethysmography System for use in Clinical & Occupational Medicine*, Medical Instrumentation, Vol. 13, #4, July/August 1979.

60. *When the Workplace is The Etiology*, Patient Care, March 1, 1977.
61. Whorton, Donald, et al., *Testicular Function in DBCP Exposed Pesticide Workers*, Journal of Occupational Medicine, Vol. 21, # 3, March 1979.
62. *Workers' Rights Under OSHA*; U.S. Department of Labor, OSHA, 1977.
63. Zim, Marvin M., *Allied Chemical's $20 Million Ordeal with Kepone*, Fortune, September 11, 1978.

Index

Acetates, 63t
Acetic acid, 51t, 59t
Acetonitrile, 64t
ACGIH. *See* American Committee of Government and Industrial Hygienists
Acids and alkalis, 51t
Acrylamide, 51t, 63t, 111t
Acrylonitrile, 32t, 38-39, 51t, 55t, 64t, 111t, 115t, 124t
ACSH. *See* American Council on Science and Health
Aesthesiometers, 140
AFL-CIO, 10
Agricultural services, forestry, fisheries, 145t, 154t
Air atmospheres, compressed, 111t
Air Shields, 110, 204
Alcoholism, 26
Alcohols, 63t
Aldrin, 32t
Alkanes, 51t, 63t, 111t
All industries, 145t
Allyl alcohol, 51t, 59t
Allyl chloride, 64t, 111t, 124t
Aluminum, 43, 127t, 131t
American Biomedical, 210
American Cancer Society, 195
American Committee of Government and Industrial Hygienists (ACGIH), 10, 11
American Council on Science and Health (ACSH), 43
American Cyanamid, 40
American Cystoscope Makers, 204
American Enterprise Institute, 14

American Journal of Industrial Medicine, 201
American Medical Association, 71, 74
American Monitor, 204
American National Standards Institute (ANSI), 9, 10, 11, 12
American Occupational Medicine Association, 5
American Optical, 137, 204
American Petroleum Institute, 97
American Thoracic Society, 110
Ames, Dr., 66
Amines, simple, 59t
4-Aminobiphenyl, 32t
Ammonia, 51t, 59t, 111t
Amyl alcohol, 51t
Anesthetics, 193, 195
Aniline, 51t
ANSI. *See* American National Standards Institute
Antimony, 43, 51t, 59t, 62t, 64t, 115t, 127t, 131t
Apparel and other textile products, 112-113t, 116-117t, 120-121t, 128-129t, 132-133t, 138-139t, 145t, 155-161t, 163-170t, 171, 173t, 174
Applied Medical Research, 204
Argosy Manufacturing, 204
Arsenic, 38, 43, 51t, 55t, 63t, 64t, 111t, 115t, 124t, 127t, 131t
Arsine, 63t, 64t
Asbestos, 10, 12, 13, 31, 32, 34-35, 54, 111t, 115t, 124t
  litigation and, 99-100
Asbestosis, 13, 34

231

Asphalt fumes, 51t, 59t, 111t
Audiometer Corporation of America, 204
Audiometry. *See* Hearing tests
Auramine, 32t
AVIV Associates, 204

Banking, 193, 194t. *See also* Finance, insurance and real estate services
Bausch & Lomb, 137, 204
Behavioral disorders, 90
Beltone Electronics, 119, 205
Benzene, 12, 18, 32t, 36-37, 51t, 54, 59t, 60t, 64t, 124t, 127t
Benzidine, 32t, 131t
Benzoyl peroxide, 51t, 59t, 111t, 124t
Benzyl chloride, 47, 51t, 111t, 115t
Beryllium, 32t, 45-46, 51t, 55t, 59t, 64t, 111t, 115t, 124t, 127t, 131t
Beryllium Case Registry, 46
Biological hazards, 22
Bio-Science Laboratories, 210
Bis (chlomethyl) ether, 55t
Bismuth, 64t, 127t, 131t
Black lung disease. *See* Pneumoconiosis
Bladder cancer, 58
Blood tests, 123-130
Boden, Les, 12, 14, 16
Boron hydrides, 51t
Boron trifluoride, 59t, 111t
BOSH. *See* Bureau of Occupational Safety and Health
Brain tumors, 57
Brass, 51t
Breath tests, 140
Breon Laboratories, 110, 205
Bromine and hydrogen bromide, 51t, 59t
Bromoform, 64t
Brown-lung disease. *See* Byssinosis
Buchler Instruments, 205
Burdick Corporation, 205
Bureau of Occupational Safety and Health (BOSH), 11
Bureau of Radiological Health, 85, 97
Business, 149t
Byssinosis, 17, 49, 58, 60

Cadmium, 32t, 43, 44, 55t, 59t, 64t, 111t, 124t, 127t, 131t
Calcium, 127t, 131t
Cambridge, Instruments, 205
Cameron Medical Corporation, 210
Cancer, 25-26, 34, 35, 36, 37, 53-58
Carbaryl, 63t, 111t, 124t
Carbon, 131t
Carbon black, 32t, 51t, 55t, 62t, 111t, 115t, 124t
Carbon dioxide, 59t, 111t, 124t

Carbon disulfide, 60t, 62t, 63t, 64t
Carbon monoxide, 47, 62t, 63t, 64t, 111t, 124t, 127t
Carbon tetrabromide, 64t
Carbon tetrachloride, 32t, 54, 60t, 64t
Carcinogens, 12, 29-47, 66, 67, 90
Cardio-Pulmonary Instruments, 114, 205
Cardiovascular disease, 61-62
Cardiovascular screening products, 119, 122
Cavitron, 110, 114, 205
CDC. *See* Centers for Disease Control
CDx, 205
Centers for Disease Control, 11, 85, 127
Central nervous system disorders, 62, 63t
Chemical hazards, 19-21, 29-52
Chemical Manufacturers Association, 97
Chemicals and allied products, 112-113t, 116-117t, 120-121t, 128-129t, 132-133t, 138-139t, 145t, 148t, 155-161t, 163-170t, 176, 177-178t
Chlordecone, 16
Chlorinated naphthalene or diphenyl compounds, 51t
Chlorine, 47, 51t, 59t, 111t, 115t
Chloroethyl methyl ether, 55t
Chloroform, 32t, 54, 60t, 63t, 64t, 111t, 124t
Chloroprene, 32t, 55t, 60t, 64t, 111t, 115t
Chromates, 55t
Chromic acid, 111t
Chromium, 32t, 51t, 64t, 115t, 124t, 127t, 131t
Chromium (VI), 55t, 111t
Chrysene, 32t, 55t
Cigarette smoking and lung cancer, 58
Coal dust, 49, 50, 59t
Coal Miner Safety and Health Act, 50
Coal mining, 8
Coal tar products, 32t, 55t, 111t, 115t, 124t
Cobalt, 43, 127t, 131t
Coffee, 49
Coke oven emissions, 12, 32t, 37-38, 55t, 111t, 115t, 124t
Communication, 72t
Comptest, 67
Computers, 140-141
Consensus Conference on Screening for Lung Cancer, 56
Construction, 72t, 145-146t, 148t, 154t
Consumer goods, 148t
Copper, 43, 127t, 131t
Cost-benefit analysis, 14-15, 17-18
Cotton dust, 49-50, 111t
Cottonseed, 49
Cresol, 51t, 64t
Curtis, Carl, 12

Index

Cyanide and cyanide salts, 59t, 111t
Cyber Diagnostics, 210
Cytogenetics, 134–135
Cytology, 131, 134–135

Damon Medical Laboratories, 210
Daniels, Representative, 10
DBCP. *See* Dibromochloropropane
DDE, 41
DDT. *See* Dichlorodiphenyltrichloroethane
Delta-aminolevulinic acid, 131t
Department of Agriculture, 85, 86t
Department of Commerce, 85, 86t
Department of Defense, 85, 86t
Department of Energy (DOE), 85, 86
Department of Health and Human Services (DHHS), 66, 84–86
Department of Health, Education and Welfare, 11
Department of Housing and Urban Development, 86t
Department of Interior, 85, 86t
Department of Labor, 10
Department of Transportation, 85, 86t
DHHS. *See* Department of Health and Human Services
Diagnostic equipment and techniques, 103–142
Diamond Shamrock Health Systems, 210
Dibromochloropropane (DBCP), 32t, 43, 51t, 59t, 60t, 64t, 111t, 124t
Dichlorodiphenyltrichloroethane (DDT), 32t, 64t
Dieldrin, 32
Digilab, 206
Diisocyanates, 115t
Dimethyl sulfate, 64t
Dinitro-ortho-cresol, 51t, 63t, 111t, 124t
Dinitrophenol, 64t
Dioxane, 33t, 51t, 54, 64t, 111t, 124t
Dioxin, 43, 60t
DOE. *See* Department of Energy
Dow Chemical Company, 41, 66, 136, 141
DuPont de Nemours, E.I., 66, 136
Dusts, 48–50
Dyna Med, 206

Eckel Industries, 206
EDC, 39
Electrical and electronic equipment, 112–113t, 116–117t, 120–121t, 128–129t, 132–133t, 138–139t, 145t, 148t, 155–161t, 163–170t, 184, 186t, 187
Electrocardiographic equipment, 122
Enbionics, 210
Endocrine Laboratories, 41

Endrin, 43, 60t
Energy, 90
Environmental Health Perspectives, 96
Environmental Protection Agency (EPA), 5, 34, 42, 43, 66, 85, 86, 97, 193
Environmental Sciences Associates, 210
Environmental Sciences Association, 206
Environmental Technology, 206
Environments, harmful, 65–68
EPA. *See* Environmental Protection Agency
Epichlorohydrin, 64t, 111t, 124t
Epidemiology, 67–68
Episodic examinations, 77–78
Equipment marketing, 199t, 200–201, 202t
Esophageal cancer, 57
Ethanol, 127t
Ether, 63t
Ethylene bromide, 64t
Ethylene chlorohydrin, 64t
Ethylene dibromide, 33t, 51t, 54, 59t, 60t, 62t, 63t, 111t, 125t
Ethylene dichloride, 33t, 54, 59t, 60t, 62t, 63t, 64t, 111t, 125t
Ethylene glycol, 64t
Ethylene oxide, 33t, 39, 51t, 60t, 125t, 193
Ethylene thiourea, 33t, 60t
Ethylenimine, 54
Ethyl silicate, 64t
Exxon Corporation, 101
Eye irritants, 50–52, 61

Fabricated metal products, 112–113t, 116–117t, 120–121t, 128–129t, 132–133t, 138–139t, 145t, 148t, 155–161t, 163–170t, 181, 183t
FDA. *See* Food and Drug Administration
Federal Mine Safety and Health Amendments Act, 88
Fetal disorders 60–61
Fibrotic and Immunologic Pulmonary Diseases Program, 58
Fibrous glass, 51t, 59t, 111t
Finance, insurance and real estate services, 145t, 147t, 149t, 154t. *See also* Banking; Insurance
Fish and Wildlife service, 85
Fluoride, 64t, 111t, 127t, 131t
Fluorocarbon decomposition products, 111t
Food and Drug Administration (FDA), 66, 85
Food and kindred products, 112–113t, 116–117t, 120–121t, 128–129t, 132–133t, 138–139t, 145t, 148t, 155–161t, 163–170t, 171, 172t
Formaldehyde, 59t, 111t

Frost & Sullivan questionnaire, 5, 217-219
Frost & Sullivan/(F&S) survey, 5, 70-71,
    73t, 75, 81-82, 104, 105, 107-108, 109,
    118, 119, 122, 123, 127, 130, 134, 137,
    141, 143, 144, 148t, 149t, 153, 171,
    172t, 174-175, 176, 177t, 179, 180t,
    181, 182-183t, 184, 185-186t, 187,
    188t, 189, 190t, 192t, 193, 195-197,
    198-199t, 200-201, 202t
  contributors to, 221-225
  geographical distribution, 150-153t
F&S survey. *See* Frost & Sullivan survey
Furniture and fixtures, 112-113t,
    116-117t, 120-121t, 128-129t,
    132-133t, 138-139t, 145t, 148t,
    155-161t, 163-170t

Gases, 19-20, 47-48
Gastrointestinal tract, cancer of, 58
General Dynamics, 101
Genetic predisposition, 25-26, 58, 61
Genie Audio, 206
George Koch Sons, 206
Glycidyl ethers, 33t, 47, 52t, 60t
Gold, 127t, 131t
Government, 149t
  Federal, 72t
  OSH-related state, 72t
  non-OSH, 72t
Graphite dust, 59t
Grayson Stadler, 207
Guenther, Arthur, 11
Gulf & Western Applied Sciences Labs, 207

Hair analysis, 135
Halogenated hydrocarbons, 63t
Hatters, 8
Hazardous agents
  causing chemical damage, 21
  causing physical damage, 20-21
  causing physiological damage, 21
Hazelton Laboratories, 41
Health Evaluation Programs, 210
Hearex Occupational Health Services, 211
Hearing tests, 118-119, 120-121t
Heat exposure, chronic, 64t, 111t
Heat stroke, 64t
Hematological tests. *See* Blood tests
Herbicide screen, 131t
Heptachlor, 33t
Herbicides, general, 40, 42-43, 60t
Hexachlorophene (HCP), 60t, 193
HLA. *See* Human leukocyte antigen
Holter monitoring, 119, 122
Hospitals, 193, 195
HSC Services, 211
Human leukocyte antigen (HLA), 26

Hydrazines, 33t, 39, 52t, 64t, 115t, 125t
Hydrogen cyanide, 47, 63t
Hydrogen fluoride, 47, 52t, 59t, 111t,
    125t
Hydrogen sulfide, 47, 52t, 59t, 63t, 111t,
    125t
Hydroquinone, 52t
Hypersusceptibility testing, 136

ICN Medical Laboratories, 211
Indium, 43, 127t, 131t
Industrial Acoustics, 207
Industrial hygienists, 73t, 75
Industrial Medicine Association, 74
Industry programs, 100-101
Inhalation Toxicology Section, 58
Injury tax, 14
Institute of Toxicology, 66
Instruments and related products,
    112-113t, 116-117t, 120-121t,
    128-129t, 132-133t, 138-139t, 145t,
    148t, 155-161t, 163-170t
Insurance, 72t, 193, 194t. *See also* Finance,
    insurance and real estate services
Iodine, 127t
IPCO, 207
Iron, 43, 127t, 131t
Iron oxide, 55t
Isopropyl alcohol, 33t, 111t, 125t
Isopropyl oil, 33t

Job Safety and Health, 98
Jobst Institute, 207
Johns Manville, 100
Johnson, Lyndon, 9
Jones Medical Instrument Company, 110,
    114, 207
Journal of Occupational Medicine, 201

Keltron Corporation, 211
Kepone, 3, 33t, 42-43, 63t, 125t
Ketones, 46, 63t, 64t, 125t
Keystone View, 137, 207
Kidney disease, 62, 64t

Laboratory Services, 211
Laboratory tests, 35, 122-136
Labor unions, 7, 12, 99-100
Lead, 33t, 44-45, 55t, 60t, 62t, 63t,
    64t, 125t, 127t, 130, 131t
Leather and leather products, 112-113t,
    116-117t, 120-121t, 128-129t,
    132-133t, 138-139t, 145t, 155-161t,
    163-170t
Leukemia, 37, 54
Lithium, 43, 127t
Litton Industries, 66

Index

Liver
  cancer of, 58
  disorders, 62, 64t
  function evaluations, 136
LSE Corporation, 110, 114, 208
Lumber and wood products, 112–113t, 116–117t, 120–121t, 128–129t, 132–133t, 138–139t, 145t, 155–161t, 163–170t, 174–175
Lung, 114–115, 134
Lung cancer, 55–57, 134
Lung function tests, 108–114

Machinery, except electrical, 112–113t, 116–117t, 120–121t, 128–129t, 132–133t, 138–139t, 145t, 148t, 155–161t, 163–170t, 184, 185t, 187
Magenta, 33t
Magnesium, 43, 127t, 131t
Maico Hearing Instruments, 119, 208
Malathion, 63t, 111t, 125t
Manganese, 43, 63t, 64t, 127t, 131t
Manufacturing, 72t, 145t, 146t, 150–151t, 153, 154t, 155–164t
Marion Health & Safety, 208
Massachusetts General Hospital, 46
Medical screening, 54, 70–71, 81–82, 103–142
Medical services, 162t, 178t, 191t, 194t. *See also* Services
  screening, 198t
Medical surveillance, 4, 69–82
  regimens, 105t
  standards, 34, 35, 37, 38, 39, 42, 44–45, 46, 47, 48, 49–50, 55
  techniques, 75–78
Medical tests, 105t, 106t
  performer of, 107t
Mediscan, 211
Mendeloff, John, 13
Mental problems, work related, 26–27
Mercury, 8, 43, 44, 60t, 63t, 64t, 125t, 127t, 131t
Mesothelioma, 57
Metals, 43–46
Methyl alcohol, 52t, 64t
Methyl bromide, 47
Methyl chloride, 64t, 111t
4,4'-Methylene-bis, 33t, 115t, 125t
Methylene chloride, 63t, 125t
Methyl parathion, 63t, 111t, 125t
Metpath, 211
Micronetic Laboratories, 211
Microwave radiation, 24–25, 52t
Mineral dust, 59t
Mining, 72t, 146t, 148t, 154t
Mining (oil and gas), 145t

Miscellaneous manufacturing industries, 112–113t, 116–117t, 120–121t, 128–129t, 132–133t, 138–139t, 145t, 155–161t, 163–170t
Mobilhealth Detection Office, 212
Molybdenum, 127t, 131t
Monitoring, of safety standards, 16
Monsanto, 43, 66
Mustard gas, 55t
Mutagens, 29–47, 60–61, 67, 91
Mycotoxins, 41

Nader, Ralph, 7, 10
Najarian, Thomas, 23
Naphthalene, 64t
Nasal cancer, 57
National Academy of Sciences, 25
National Aeronautics and Space Administration, 85, 86t
National Bureau of Standards, 85
National Cancer Institute (NCI), 39, 56, 66, 84, 96
National Draeger, 208
National Eye Institute (NEI), 85
National Heart, Lung and Blood Institute (NHLBI), 58, 84, 96
National Institute for Occupational Safety and Health (NIOSH), 3, 11, 12, 30, 31, 39, 42, 46, 47, 48, 54, 57, 66, 75, 76, 80, 85, 86–90, 99, 101, 108, 118, 136, 140, 143
National Institute for Occupational Safety and Health (NIOSH) survey, 5, 71, 72t, 74–75, 104–105, 106t, 107, 109, 112–113t, 118, 119, 120–121t, 122, 123, 128–129t, 130, 132–133, 134, 137, 138–139t, 143, 144, 145t, 147t, 153, 162t, 163–170t, 171, 174, 176, 178t, 179, 181, 184, 187, 189, 191t, 193, 194t, 195–197
National Institute of Allergy and Infectious Diseases (NIAID), 85
National Institute of Arthritis, Diabetes, and Digestive and Kidney Diseases (NIADDKD), 85
National Institute of Environmental Health Sciences (NIEHS), 41, 58, 66, 84, 91–96, 99
National Institute of General Medical Sciences (NIGMS), 84
National Institute of Neurological and Communicative Disorders and Stroke (NINCDS), 84–85
National Institutes of Health (NIH), 84–85
National Library of Medicine, 85
National Science Foundation, 85, 86t

National Toxicology Program, 66
NCI. See National Cancer Institute
NEI. See National Eye Institute
Neurological disorders, 137, 140
NHLBI. See National Heart, Lung and Blood Institute
NIADDKD. See National Institute of Arthritis, Diabetes, and Digestive and Kidney Diseases
NIAID. See National Institute of Allergy and Infectious Diseases
Nickel, 33t, 43, 52t, 55t, 111t, 127t, 131t
Nickel carbonyl, 33t, 111t, 115t, 125t
NIEHS. See National Institute of Environmental Health Sciences
NIGMS. See National Institute of General Medical Sciences
NIH. See National Institutes of Health
NINCDS. See National Institute of Neurological and Communicative Disorders and Stroke
NIOSH. See National Institute for Occupational Safety and Health
Nitric acid, 111t
Nitriles, 59t, 62t, 63t, 64t, 111t, 115t
Nitrobenzene, 64t
4-Nitrodiphenyl, 33t
Nitrogen dioxide, 47, 48
Nitrogen oxides, 59t, 111t
Nitroglycerin, 62t
Nitrous oxide, 47, 48, 55t, 193, 195
Nixon, Richard, 10, 11
Noise, 22-23, 119
Nuclear plants, 148t
Nuclear Regulatory Commission, 85, 86t, 97
Nurses, 73t, 74-75

Occupational Health & Safety, 201
Occupational illness, 3
Occupational injury, 3, 13
Occupational medicine
  defined, 71
  federal government and, 84-99
  history, 8-9
  marketplace, 143-202
  personnel, 71-75
  training in, 99
Occupational Safety and Health Act, 3, 10
Occupational Safety and Health Administration (OSHA), 3, 7-8, 10-11, 30-31, 34, 36, 37, 38, 42, 44, 47, 49-50, 55, 70, 74, 76, 77, 78-80, 88, 96-98, 101, 104, 119, 130, 131, 141, 143, 144, 171, 193
  Regional offices, 215
Office of Research and Technology, 85
Ohio Medical Products, 110, 208

Oil, Chemical, and Atomic Workers Union, 10, 12
Ophthalmological screening, 136-137, 138-139t
Oral cancer, 57
Ordnance and accessories, 145t
Organic dusts, 59t
Organophosphates, 127t, 131t
Organotin compounds, 52t, 62t, 63t, 64t, 115t, 125t
Oryzalin, 43
OSHA. See Occupational Safety and Health Administration
O-Tolidine, 33t
Oxalic acid, 64t
Ozone, 47, 48, 59t, 111t, 115t

Pacific Southwest Medical Group, 212
PAH. See Polycyclic aromatic hydrocarbons
Palladium, 43
Pancreas, cancer of, 57
Paper and allied products, 112-113t, 116-117t, 120-121t, 128-129t, 132-133t, 138-139t, 145t, 148t, 155-161t, 163-170t, 174-175
Parasitology Laboratory of Washington, 212
Parathion, 63t, 125t, 127t
Park Surgical Co., 208
PBB. See Polybrominated biphenyls
PCB. See Polychlorinated biphenyls
Periodic examinations, 77
Pesticides, general, 33t, 40, 42-43, 60t, 63t, 125t
Petroleum, 36-37
  solvent, refined, 59t, 111t, 126t
Petroleum and coal products, 112-113t, 116-117t, 120-121t, 128-129t, 132-133t, 138-139t, 145t, 148t, 155-161t, 163-170t, 179, 180t
Phenol, 52t, 63t, 64t, 111t, 125t, 127t, 131t
Phenylhydrazine, 64t
Phone-A-Gram System, 212
Phosgene, 59t, 111t, 115t
Phosphorus, 43
  yellow, 64t
Physical hazards, 22-25
Physical Measurements, 212
Physicians, 71, 73t, 74
Physio-Control, 208
Picker Corporation, 208
Plant products, 52t
Platinum, 43
Plethysmography, 140
Pneumoconiosis, 50
Polybrominated biphenyls (PBB), 41
Polychlorinated biphenyls (PCB), 33t, 41, 52t, 60t, 64t, 126t

Index

Polycyclic aromatic hydrocarbons (PAH), 36, 37
Polyvinyl chloride (PVC), 35
Potassium, 127t
Pregnancy, 60–61
Preplacement examination, 76
Pressure, 25
Pretoxic indicators, 76–77
Preventive medicine, 16–17, 81–82
Primary metal industries, 112–113t, 116–117t, 120–121t, 128–129t, 132–133t, 138–139t, 145t, 148t, 155–161t, 163–170t, 181, 182t
Printing and publishing, 112–113t, 116–117t, 120–121t, 128–129t, 132–133t, 138–139t, 145t, 148t, 155–161t, 163–170t
Privacy Protection Study Commission, 80
Proctor & Gamble, 66
Products market, 199t, 200
 suppliers, 203–209
Professional Health Services, 212
Propylene dichloride, 64t
Prostate, cancer of, 57
Protoporphyrin, 127, 130
Public Health Service, 45
Pulmonary function testing equipment, 110
PVC. *See* Polyvinyl chloride
Pyridine, 64t

Radiation, 23–25
 nonionizing, health effects of, 24t
Radon, 55t, 189
Reagan, Ronald, 15, 17
Record keeping, 78–81
Reedco, 209
Regulation, 96–98
Reproductive disorders, 60–61, 90
Reproductive function evaluations, 135
Research, government, 84–96
Research Triangle Institute, 41
Respiratory disease, 58–60, 90
Roswell Park Memorial Institute, 54
Rubber and plastics products, 112–113t, 116–117t, 120–121t, 128–129t, 132–133t, 138–139t, 145t, 148t, 155–161t, 163–170t

Saccade velocity measurement, 137
Safety standards, 12
Sales, 154t
Screening
 installations, 141–142
 programs, 103–142
Selenium, 43, 64t, 127t, 131t
Selikoff, Irving, M.D., 9
Services, 72t, 145t, 147t, 154t, 189–195.
 See also Medical services
 markets, 196–197, 198t
 suppliers, 203, 210–212
Silica, 49, 55t, 111t, 115t
Silver, 43, 127t, 131t
Skin irritants, 50–52, 62
Smith, Robert, 14
Smith Kline Diagnostics, 209
Smith & Wesson, 209
Snell, Foster D., 144
Sodium, 127t
Sodium hydroxide, 59t, 111t
Solvents, 38–39, 46–47, 52t
Spirometers, 110, 114
Sputum cytology, 134
SRL Medical, 110, 209
Stauffer Chemical, 66
Steiger, William, 10
Sterility, in men, 61
Stilbene, 63t
Stone, clay and glass products, 112–113t, 116–117t, 120–121t, 128–129t, 132–133t, 138–139t, 145t, 148t, 155–161t, 163–170t
Stress, 26–27, 61, 62, 90, 119, 122, 193
Styrene, 63t, 64t
Styrene butadiene, 33t
Sulfur dioxide, 47–48, 59t, 111t
Sulfuric acid, 59t, 111t
Sulfur oxide, 52t
Supreme Court, 17–18
Synthetic resins, 52t

2, 4, 5-T. *See* 2, 4, 5-Trichlorophenoxy-acetic acid
TCDD. *See* 2, 3, 7, 8-Tetrachlorodibenzo-p-dioxin
Tellurium, 127t, 131t
Temperature, 25
Teratogens, 40–41, 60–61, 67, 91
p-Tert-butyltoluene, 46
Testing equipment, 108t
 new developments, 108
Testing regimens, 172–173t, 175t, 177t, 180t, 182–183t, 185–186t, 188t, 190t, 192t
1,1,2,2-Tetrachloroethane, 54, 63t, 64t, 126t
Tetrachloroethylene, 54, 59t, 60t, 62t, 63t, 64t, 111t, 126t
2,3,7,8-Tetrachlorodibenzo-p-dioxin (TCDD), 43
Textile Manufacturer's Association, 97
Textile mill products, 112–113t, 116–117t, 120–121t, 128–129t, 132–133t, 138–139t, 145t, 148t, 155–161t, 163–170t, 171, 173t, 174
Textiles, 8
Thallium, 43, 127t, 131t

Thiols, 52t, 63t, 126t
Tin, 131t
Tissue analysis, 135
Titmus Optical, 137, 209
Tobacco products, 112-113t, 116-117t, 120-121t, 128-129t, 132-133t, 138-139t, 145t, 148t, 155-161t, 163-170t, 171, 172t
Toluene, 47, 63t, 64t, 126t, 127t, 131t
Toluene diisocyanate, 52t, 59t, 111t, 115t, 126t
Tonometry, 136, 137
TOSCA. *See* Toxic Substances Control Act
Toxaphene, 40
Toxic substances, 21, 41-42, 62
  classification of, 30-31
Toxicology, 66-67
Toxic Substances Control Act (TOSCA), 5, 66, 88
ToxiGenics, 212
Tracor, 209
Trades, 72t
Transportation, 72t, 154t
Transportation and other public utilities, 145t, 147t
Transportation equipment, 112-113t, 116-117t, 120-121t, 128-129t, 132-133t, 138-139t, 145t, 148t, 155-161t, 163-170t, 187, 188t
TRC, The Research Group Corp. of New England, 212
1,1,1-Trichloroethane, 54, 63t, 64t, 111t, 126t
Trichloroethylene, 46, 54, 63t, 64t, 111t, 126t, 131t
2,4,5-Trichlorophenoxyacetic acid (2,4,5-T), 43
Trimellitic anhydride, 59t
Tungsten, 43
Tungsten and cemented tungsten carbide, 52t, 111t, 115t

UBTL Division, 212
Union Carbide, 101
United Automobile Workers, 10
United Rubberworkers, 12
Uranium, 55t, 64t
Urinalysis, 130, 131t, 132-133t
Urinary cytology, 134
Utilities, 72t, 149t, 189, 190-191t

Vanadium, 52t, 59t, 111t, 115t, 127t, 131t
Veterans' Administration, 85, 86t
Vibration, 25, 64t, 137, 140
Vinyl bromide, 33t
Vinyl chloride, 12, 33t, 35-36, 55t, 126t
Vinyl halides, 33t
Vital Assists, 209
Vitalograph Medical Instrumentation, 110, 209
Vocational Rehabilitation Act, 26

Walsh-Healey Act, 9, 13
Warren E. Collins, 110, 114, 206
Waste anesthetic gases and vapors, 60t
Wegman, David, 12, 14, 16
Weidenbaum, Murray, 15
Wholesale and retail trade, 145t, 147t
Williams, Harrison, 10
Williams-Steiger, 10, 11, 97
Workers, without medical examinations, 145t

X-rays, 114-118
Xylene, 59t, 63t, 111t, 126t, 127t, 131t

Yale Medical School, 60
Yasbin, Dr. Ronald, 67

Zeranol, 41
Zinc, 43, 127t, 131t
Zinc oxide, 111t

NO LONGER THE PROPERTY
OF THE
UNIVERSITY OF R.I. LIBRARY